# Down's syndrome. Psychological, psychobiological, and socio-educational perspectives.

# Down's syndrome. Psychological, psychobiological, and socio-educational perspectives.

Edited by

Jean A. Rondal,

Juan Perera,

Lynn Nadel,

and Annick Comblain

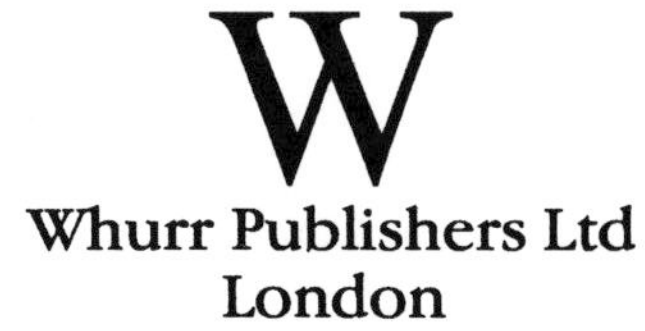

Whurr Publishers Ltd
London

First published 1996 by
Whurr Publishers Ltd
19b Compton Terrace, London N1 2UN, England



**British Library Cataloguing-in-Publication Data**
A catalogue record for this book is available from the British Library.

ISBN: 1-897635-09-5

Printed and bound in the UK by Athenaeum Press Ltd,
Gateshead, Tyne & Wear.

# Contents

# Preface

This book came out of an International Symposium devoted to the Psychology and Psychobiology, Educational, and Social integration of Down's syndrome persons co-organized by Juan Perera and Jean A. Rondal. It took place at the Club Diario in Palma de Mallorca, Baleares, Spain, 24–26 February 1995. The symposium was placed under the high auspices of the Govern Balear, the Real Patronato de Prevenciòn y de Atenciòn a Personas con Minusvalìa, INSERSO (Instituto Nacional de Servicios Sociales), the Universidad de Las Islas Baleares, EDSA (European Down Syndrome Association), FEISD (Federaciòn Española de Instituciones para el Sìndrome de Down), and ASNIMO (Associaciòn Sìndrome de Down de Baleares).

The organizers are pleased to acknowledge the following sponsorship to the symposium: Department of Health and Social Security, Balearic Government; Department of Culture, Education and Sport, Balearic Government; the Council of the Island of Mallorca; the Palma Town Council; the Provincial Directorate of the National Institute of Social Services; the Balearic Savings Bank 'sa Nostra'; the UNAC (Balearic Islands' Union of Association and Centres of Assistance for the Disabled); the Diario of Mallorca Newspaper; the Ultima Hora Newspaper; the Groups Sol, Riu; and the Hotel Bon Sol.

The lectures to the Palma Symposium by a number of distinguished and internationally recognized colleagues have been reworked and adapted to book publication under the editorial supervision of Jean A Rondal, Juan Perera, Lynn Nadel, and Annick Comblain. We wish to express our gratitude to the following people who helped at various stages of the editorial work: Carmen Crespo, María Rosa Pizà, Maribel Liébana, María García, Anastasia Piat-Di Nicolantonio, Brigitte Théwis, and Mercedes George. Lastly, we should like to acknowledge the professional courtesy of Illustration Unlimited, L.V. Kibiuck, Baltimore, for authorizing the reproduction of Figure 1.1, in K. Wiesniewski *et al.*'s chapter, and Paul H. Brooks, Publishing Co., Baltimore, for authorizing the reproduction and adaption of Figure 13.1 in D. Van Dyke *et al.*'s chapter.

# Contributors

**M Beveridge** School of Education, Bristol University, UK.

**G Bird** Sarah Duffen Centre & Department of Psychology, University of Portsmouth, Southsea, UK.

**W Ted Brown** Medical Research Centre, Polish Academy of Science, Warsaw, Poland.

**S Buckley** Sarah Duffen Centre & Department of Psychology, University of Portsmouth, Southsea, UK.

**A Byrne** Sarah Duffen Centre & Department of Psychology, University of Portsmouth, Southsea, UK.

**I G Candel** ASSIDO (Murcia) and Faculty of Education, University of Murcia, Spain.

**J A Carranza Carnicero** Faculty of Education, University of Murcia, Spain.

**S Clarke** Department of Psychology, University of Southampton, Southampton, UK.

**A Comblain** Psycholinguistic Laboratory, University of Liège, Belgium.

**M J Guralnick** Child Development and Mental Retardation Center, University of Washington, Seattle, USA.

**R Hodapp** Graduate School of Education, University of California, Los Angeles, USA

**E Kida** Health Science Center, State University of New York, Brooklyn, New York, USA.

**P J Mattheis** University Hospital School Division of Developmental Disabilities, The University of Iowa, Iowa City, USA.

**D M McBrien** University Hospital School, Division of Developmental Disabilities, The University of Iowa, Iowa City, USA.

**B Myers** Rhode Island Hospital , Brown University School of Medicine, Providence, Rhode Island, USA.

**L Nadal** Department of Psychology, University of Arizona, Tucson, USA.

**J Perera** ASNIMO (Palma de Mallorca) and University of the Baleares Palma de Mallorca, Spain.

**J Pérez López** Faculty of Education, University of Murcia, Spain.

**S M Pueschel** Rhode Island Hospital, Brown University School of Medicine, Providence, Rhode Island, USA.

**R Remington** Department of Psychology, University of Southampton, Southampton, UK.

**J A Rondal** Psycholinguistic Laboratory, University of Liège, Belgium.

**W Silverman** Institute for Basic Research in Developmental Disabilities, State Island, New York, USA.

**M Sustrova** Institute of Preventive and Clinical Medicine, Bratislava, Slovak Republic.

**D C Van Dyke** University Hospital School Division of Developmental Disabilities, The University of Iowa, Iowa City, USA.

**J Wishart** Moray House Institute of Education, Heriot-Watt University, Edinburgh, UK.

**H M Wisniewski** Institute for Basic Research in Developmental Disabilities, Staten Island, New York, USA.

**K E Wisniewski** Institute for Basic Research in Developmental Disabilities, Staten Island, New York, USA.

# Introduction

The main objective of the Palma Symposium, reflected in this book, was to propose a state-of-the-art review and analysis of a number of aspects of the psychobiology, psychology, education and social integration of individuals with Down's syndrome (DS). Accordingly, the book's fifteen chapters have been divided into six sections: (1) Psychobiology; (2) Perception and cognition; (3) Language and communication; (4) Early intervention; (5) Personality and development; and (6) Integration.

In Chapter 1, K Wisniewski, Kida, and Brown analyse the immediate consequences of the genetic abnormalities in DS on brain structures, particularly the neuropathological and immunocytochemical changes. They review prenatal, perinatal and postnatal brain development, including the hippocampal abnormalities observed. Nadel, in Chapter 2, discusses aspects of learning and memory in individuals with DS in a framework provided by the analysis of the neural systems known to underlie these functions. He specifies some of the major neural sequellae of DS in a lifespan perspective, from birth onto adulthood and ageing, with particular regard to cognitive functions. In Chapter 3, H Wisniewski and Silverman summarize present knowledge on clinical and neuropathological aspects of Alzheimer's disease (AD), the most common cause of old-age associated dementia in normal people, to which adults with DS are particularly vulnerable.

Pueschel and Sustrova, in Chapter 4, review and summarize the literature on visual and auditory sensory processing and perception in DS individuals. Two more chapters map the domain of cognitive development and functioning in DS persons. In Chapter 5, Hodapp discusses the important question of how development is organized in DS. He devotes several pages to analysing previous and current theoretical positions on the so-called delay-difference issue in mental retardation and DS. This issue has been reformulated in terms of the similar sequence and similar structure hypothesis and Hodapp discusses its status across cognitive domains. In Chapter 6, Wishart analyses data concerned with the way DS children approach the task of learning, including motivational aspects. She devotes several pages to reviewing developmental trends in operant learning and object concept development in DS infants.

Three chapters are devoted to language and communication in DS. In Chapter 7, Rondal supplies a comprehensive picture of spoken language development in DS children and language functioning in DS adolescents and adults. He discusses the issue of the existence of a critical period for some aspects of language development in DS individuals and the implications of this finding for language remediation. The question of the large inter-individual variability in DS individuals' language is also dealt with, including the mention of the existence of exceptional cases of language development in DS, and the implications of these findings for theoretical questions such as the modular nature of oral language. In Chapter 8, Buckley, Bird and Byrne, argue for the usefulness of early literacy training in children with DS. They discuss appropriate teaching methods, the DS children's reading strategies, and the benefits of literacy training for spoken language development and structuring, as well as for other cognitive skills. Remington and Clarke, in Chapter 9, analyse types of alternative and augmentative systems of communication (AAC) that can be used with DS individuals. They conclude that several AAC systems (for instance, those based on sign gestures) are appropriate for DS individuals under some conditions. In Chapter 10, Guralnick specifies future directions for early intervention with DS children. The effects of early intervention on intellectual development are analysed together with peer-related social competence and family processes.

Candel, Carranza Carnicero and Pérez López, in Chapter 11, discuss the available data on socio-effective development and temperamental variables in DS infants and children. Chapter 12 by Pueschel, Myers and Sustrova, is on psychiatric disorders in persons with DS. A wide range of psychopathology in DS adults is noted including obsessive compulsive disorders, anorexia, phobias, etc. Behavioural observations relating to these disorders are analysed and assessment procedures are reviewed. In Chapter 13, Van Dyke, McBrien and Mattheis review and discuss studies and current positions and practices relating to psychosexual behaviour and management issues in individuals with DS. They analyse the medical aspects of male and female sexuality in DS and deal with a series of difficult issues such as sexual abuse, contraception, pregnancy, marriage, parenting and HIV infection in persons with DS. It is reaffirmed that individuals with DS have the right to develop and express their sexuality in an emotionally satisfying and socially appropriate manner.

The last two chapters are devoted to integration issues. In Chapter 14, Beveridge discusses school policies and integration processes, as well as the particular problems raised in the case of DS pupils at various levels of the school curriculum. The need for teachers' support is acknowledged and technical questions, such as pupil ratios, are discussed. Attitudes to integration and social learning are also analysed. In Chapter 15, Perera deals with social and labour integration of DS adults and the question how best to prepare these adults for work. A series of work alternatives are envisaged that include occupational centres, protected workshops, special employment centres, employment with support, small businesses, etc. It is stressed that labour integration is the key to social integration and personal maturity.

A series of concluding comments terminates the book. They embody current perspectives on the treatment of Down's syndrome and its lifespan management, and reaffirm the necessity to envisage Down's syndrome according to its most specific aspects.

# Part One: Psychobiology

# Chapter 1 Consequences of Genetic Abnormalities in Down's Syndrome on Brain Structure and Function

KRYSTYNA E WISNIEWSKI, ELZBIETA KIDA AND W TED BROWN

## 1.1 Introduction

As a result of having an extra chromosome 21, and the consequent abnormal gene dosage, structural and functional abnormalities occur in the central nervous system (CNS) which result in varying degrees of cognitive and other neurological dysfunction in children with Down's syndrome (DS). Impaired differentiation and maturation of the CNS brain associated with a mild degree of cortical dysplasia results in decreased numbers of neurons, abnormal synaptogenesis, and delayed brain development. These CNS abnormalities are present during the late prenatal period (Wisniewski and Kida 1995). They may be caused by abnormal differentiation and maturation due to gene dosage effects. These may alter genetic programming, or directly result in disregulation of gene expression.

At present, it is estimated that human beings have approximately 50 000–100 000 genes. Since chromosome 21 has about 1.7% of the genetic material, there are an estimated 850–1700 genes on chromosome 21. Approximately, 40 of these genes have been identified and mapped (McKusick 1994). Approximately 95% of DS individuals have full trisomy 21, while the remainder have either a translocation or mosaicism. Of individuals with full trisomy 21, about 5% have received a double copy of chromosome 21 from the father and a single one from the mother. For the other 95%, a double copy is derived from the mother. Of these, about 75% are because of a cell division error at meiosis I, while about 25% are due to meiosis II errors. Recently it has been determined that maternal meiosis I errors involve a maternal age-dependent mechanism, which is associated with only about one third of the expected rate of recombination between the two chromatids

(Sherman *et al.* 1994). Meiosis II errors would result in a double copy of a single chromosome 21, derived either from the mother's mother or her father. Differential activity of genomic regions depending on the parent of origin, known as 'genomic imprinting,' has recently been recognized as playing a role in several human genetic conditions. Genomic imprinting effects resulting from uniparental disomy of human chromosome 21 may also play a role in the DS phenotype (Henderson *et al.* 1994). Korenberg *et al.* (1994) have suggested that the pheno- and genotype in DS may be considered to be that of a contiguous gene syndrome. Her studies provide evidence that genes located at various chromosome 21 locations contribute to the DS phenotype, including the characteristic facial features, microcephaly, short stature, abnormal dermatoglyphics, hypotonia, mental retardation and cognitive dysfunction.

The specific genes responsible for the brain abnormalities causing different degrees of cognitive dysfunction in DS children are still unknown. However, during brain development, differentiation and maturation, neurons are subject to programmed cell death (PCD), or 'apoptosis', which is under tight genetic control. The genetic basis of PCD is well characterized in several model organisms, such as the roundworm, ***Caenorhabditis elegans***, but not yet in humans (Yuan and Horvitz 1990; Hengartner *et al.* 1992). It has been determined that in both worms and humans many more neurons are formed than are ultimately required, and as a result, a huge number of surplus neurons and glia cells undergo PCD. In ***Caenorhabditis elegans*** all of the 1090 cells that appear during the worm's embryonic development have been specifically identified; 131 of them are known to die in a programmed way as the worm matures. Mortality and vitality appear to depend on the presence of killer genes, ced-3-4, and lifesaver genes, ced-9, which have opposite effects. In human studies, a gene involved with cellular survival bcl-2 (B cell lymphoma/leukaemia 2) has been expressed in cultured neurons (Garcia *et al.* 1992). Bcl-2 keeps cells from dying even in the absence of nerve growth factor (NGF), which normally also prevents cell death. We have recently identified prenatally increased bcl-2 immunoreactivity in DS fetuses at 20-24 weeks gestational age (WGA) suggesting abnormal differentiation and maturation in DS (Wisniewski and Kida 1995).

It has been found that genetic programming of development in vertebrates occurs largely under the control of a set of master genes termed 'homeobox genes'. These genes specify cell identity along the anterior–posterior axis of the embryo. They spell out how and when the structure of different cell types should form and which cells are assigned to new locations to form organs. The deoxyribonucleic acid (DNA) sequences found in these classes of genes are evolutionarily highly related and direct the development of body structure in virtually all animals, including worms, flies, birds, mice and humans (Ruddle *et al.* 1994). Since the homeobox genes have remained very similar during millions of years of evolution in many species, biologists suspect their sequences are essential to life. The function of these genes is to encode proteins that can bind to DNA in such a way that they turn other genes on or off. A subset of the homeobox genes are termed 'HOX genes'. They are lined up in four clusters on chromosomes 2, 7, 12, 17. The linear arrangement of these genes that control the morphogenesis parallels that of the body parts, e.g., head with brain, trunk (see Figure 1.1). When the function of one of the genes is changed, abnormalities of the body parts will develop, causing birth defects.

The precise number of HOX genes differs significantly in vertebrates,

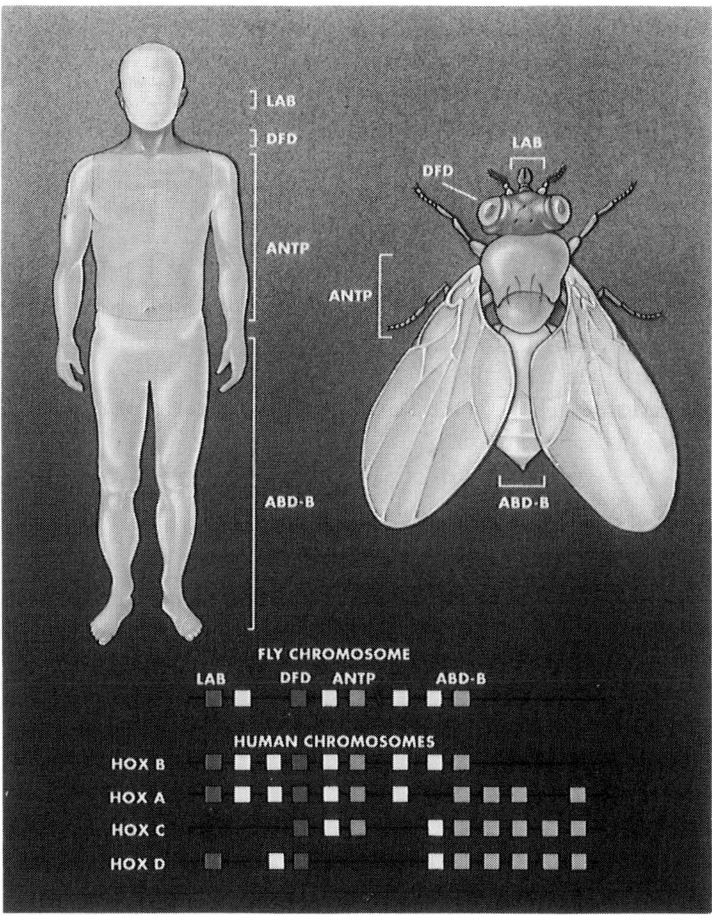


*Figure 1.1* HOX genes, which control development of the central nervous system and the body, are common to most organisms. Four groups of similar HOX genes, appear to control related regions of the human body and the fly. Each box above represents a single HOX gene. From: 'Hox genes and birth defects' in Brain Briefings, K. Wisniewski, pamphlet to the Society for Neuroscience, Washington, December 1994. Reprinted by permission.

invertebrates and humans (Zappavigna *et al.* 1991; Price *et al.* 1992; Renucci *et al.* 1992). Another class of homeobox genes are termed 'PAX genes' and also control development (Stuart *et al.* 1993). They are generally found in isolation on different chromosomes. So far, there are at least nine different PAX genes known, although none are localized to chromosome 21. Other homeobox genes are also involved in development. For example, a homeobox gene Lim1 recently has been shown to be involved in mouse head organizational development (Shawlot and Behringer 1995). There are probably many more such homeobox genes yet unidentified. Thus, it is likely that some of the genes on chromosome 21 could be homeobox genes or homeobox modifier genes, and their imbalance could result in abnormal brain development.

In humans at birth, when the CNS is formed, about 70-80 billion neurons are usually present (Haug 1986). They are organized into networks and regions, and some neurons have specialized functions. In the prenatal and postnatal stages of CNS development, differentiation and maturation, numerous factors such as growth, neuropeptides, cell adhesion molecules, cytokines, glutamate receptors and calcium channels also exert significant influence. Deficiency or excess of any of these factors may alter functional, biochemical and morphological events. Growth hormone and/or nerve growth factors and thyroid hormone may serve as signals for synchronization of developmental sequences. Any desynchronization of the signal or signals during critical periods of CNS maturation and differentiation leads to a series of consequences that may affect development and maturation and result in increased selective neuronal death, reduced number of neurons, abnormal synaptogenesis, impaired myelinogenesis and the Alzheimer type of pathology that is seen in DS individuals.

The brains of persons with DS have been examined and described by many authors starting at the beginning of this century (Apert 1914; Gans 1925) and have increased in number particularly in recent years (Benda 1969; Courchesne 1988; Crome *et al.* 1966; Jacob 1956; Kemper 1988; Ross *et al.* 1984; Scott *et al.* 1982, 1983; Wisniewski *et al.* 1984, 1986; Wisniewski 1990; Wisniewski and Schmidt-Sidor 1989; Wisniewski and Kida 1995). In the following sections, the neuropathological and immunocytochemical changes observed in the CNS of individuals with DS will be reviewed.

## 1.2 Prenatal and Perinatal Development

The morphogenesis of the CNS is a highly complex process. Shortly after closure, the neural tube differentiates regionally into the spinal cord and three brain vesicles: the forebrain (telencephalon and diencephalon), the midbrain (mesencephalon) and the hindbrain (metencephalon and myelencephalon) are formed. These vesicles are further subdivided into smaller regions, phylogenetically and functionally different, to give rise to what can be interpreted as segment-like structures.

Cortical development starts approximately at 4 WGA. Initially, the neuronal tube forms with a simple pseudostratified neuroepithelium, which then proliferates and continues to surround the developing ventricular system, eventually becoming the ventricular zone. Neuroblast migration then begins and by approximately 6 WGA, the ventricular zone, intermediate zone and marginal zone of the cortical mantle can be appreciated as distinct (Rorke 1994). The initial cortical plate is first noted at 7–10 WGA. A primary condensation of this cortical plate occurs as it compacts. At 11–13 WGA, a bilaminate appearance is noted in the cortical plate, followed at 13–15 WGA by a secondary condensation. At approximately 16 WGA, a condensation into six-layered cortex is noted. Neuroblasts continue to migrate through the intermediate zone (future white matter) through radial gliophilic and neurophilic paths to the cortex, a process that can continue up to a few months after birth (Sidman and Rakic 1973). Neurons of the deepest cortical layers are the first to radially migrate, while the neuroblasts destined for the more superficial cortical layers migrate past them (Angevine and Sidman 1961).

Observations concerning prenatal development of the CNS in individuals with DS are rare. Sylvester (1983) found a DS brain to be smaller and the hippocampus less mature compared to a control brain at 18 WGA. A more exhaustive morphometric study performed by Schmidt-Sidor *et al.* (1990) on 17 DS and 10 non-DS age-matched fetuses from 15–22 WGA demonstrated that during this span of time, no gross differences in brain growth and maturation are evident. In both groups, the heads of fetuses were brachycephalic, with similar circumferences and configurations of frontal and temporal lobes with almost the same size of cerebellum and brainstem. Development of the cerebral and cerebellar cortices, as far as myelination of the spinal cord and brain stem tracts, occurred at the same stage of development. Biochemical studies of the composition of gangliosides, neuronal cell adhesion molecules and the activity of acetylcholinesterase also did not indicate differences between DS and non-DS fetal brains at this stage of development (Brooksbank *et al.* 1989). Neuropathological information regarding brain weight and shape between 22–40 WGA is missing. Recently our immunocytochemical studies showed, compared with controls, a different pattern of synaptophysin immunoreactivity in the cortical mantle with disturbed cortical lamination in some DS fetuses after 20 WGA (Wisniewski and Kida 1995). Abnormal cortical lamination in the superior temporal gyri was found by Golden and Hyman (1995).

The first mild difference in brain weight between DS and non-DS groups was described at birth by Wisniewski *et al.* (1986), Wisniewski (1990) and Schmidt-Sidor *et al.* (1990). They estimated the weights of DS newborn brains to be lower than those of non-DS controls, although they could be considered in the lower normal weight range. Benda (1971) considered the weight of DS newborn brains to be nearly normal. Morphometric examination showed that neuronal densities in the occipital, temporal and frontal areas was lower in DS than non-DS subjects at birth (Wisniewski *et al.* 1984, 1986, 1993; Wisniewski 1990). The morphology of neurons, their dendrites and synaptic spines was estimated, using the Golgi-rapid method by Takashima *et al.* (1981), to be similar in both DS and non-DS brains up to 40 WGA. In contrast, at the ultrastructural level decreased synaptic density and presynaptic length, average surface area per synaptic contact and anomalies in synaptic morphology was revealed (Petit *et al.* 1984; Wisniewski *et al.* 1986). Disturbed electrical membrane properties of the fetal brain are observed very early, in the 16th WGA (Scott *et al.* 1982, 1983).

The results cited above reveal that first differences between DS and non-DS brains are observed during the second half of fetal development. The data presented by various authors, sometimes controversial, depending on the population examined and methods used for examination, prove that the degree of observed changes may be mild to moderate. Nevertheless, particular features found in the neuronal population of the cerebral cortex in newborns with DS indicate that the changes occurring so early during brain development require further research studies at the molecular and biochemical levels.

## 1.3 Postnatal Brain Development from Birth

After birth, CNS changes occurring in developing DS brains become much more evident than those observed during fetal and perinatal life and are particularly accentuated during late infancy and early childhood. In healthy individuals, brain weight is about 300 g at birth, is tripled by one year, quadrupled by four years and, sometimes, quintupled by 12 years of age. In DS, from day one, and especially after midinfancy, the brain weight is usually 10–50% lower than in individuals without DS (Wisniewski *et al.* 1986). Brain weight of mature individuals who do not have DS is usually 1200–1500 g, whereas that of individuals with DS is 700–1100 g.

Head circumference (HC) measurements of children with DS are 1 to 3 SD lower than the expected value during the first two years of age (Roche 1966), in 50% of children with DS younger than three years of age (Palmer *et al.* 1992) and in 80% younger than five years of age (Wisniewski 1990) HC remains in the normal or lower-normal range in 20% of DS children. HC of mature non-DS individuals, is usually between 50–60 cm, whereas that of DS individuals is 46–52 cm. In infants with DS, decreased brain weight parallels the increasingly evident small head. The differences in brain weight after birth between individuals with DS and persons without DS have also been observed by other authors (Wisniewski *et al.* 1986, 1990; Schmidt-Sidor *et al.* 1990). The degree of brain weight reduction in infants and children with DS compared to that of age-matched control subjects was evaluated and was statistically significant (Wisniewski *et al.* 1986). Therefore, individuals with DS can often be diagnosed as microcranial and microencephalic (Wisniewski 1990).

The shape of brains in DS observed in the majority of cases presents some characteristic features. The first one observed by many authors, shortened dimension of antero-posterior diameter, has been attributed to reduction or hypoplasia of the frontal lobes (Benda 1971; Crome and Stern 1972; Schmidt-Sidor *et al.* 1990; Wisniewski *et al.* 1986; Wisniewski 1990). However, this was not confirmed in another study (Kemper 1988).

Narrowed superior temporal gyrus (STG) in one or both hemispheres was found in 33% of cases by Schmidt-Sidor *et al.* (1990) and in 50% by Friede (1989) and Zellweger (1977) (see Figure 1.2). In individuals with DS with severe speech abnormalities (more expressive than receptive), magnetic resonance imaging (MRI) scans of the head as well as postmortem studies showed severe narrowing of the STG, with widening of the Sylvian fissure and shortening of the frontal lobes. MRI of the superior temporal-gyri and inferior frontal gyrus, where the speech centres are localized, showed abnormalities in some individuals with DS with severe speech abnormalities. Unfortunately, in these DS children even early intervention and proper education do not drastically improve speech abilities. We have found that there are more speech abnormalities in individuals with DS who had narrowing of STG bilaterally or in the dominant hemisphere. More detailed brain volume studies are in progress. The small size of the cerebellum and brainstem in people with DS as compared with individuals who do not have DS has been reported many times (Crome *et al.* 1966; Friede 1989; Gulotta and Rehder 1974; Wisniewski 1990). The ratio of the cerebellum and brainstem weights to the cerebrum weight was estimated to be 1:9 in DS and 1:7 in non-DS subjects (Crome *et al.* 1966).

Myelination was delayed in 22.5% of children with DS and in only 6.8% of children without DS. The myelination delay mainly affected tracts with late beginning and slow cycles of myelination, mainly long association and intercortical fibres of the frontal and temporal lobes. In individuals with DS, with advanced myelination, only 30% U-fibres are less myelinated. This abnormality also has an influence on associated fibres (Wisniewski and Schmidt-Sidor 1989).

Morphometric studies at the light microscopic level showed that the thickness of cortical areas 10, 17 and 28 did not significantly differ in children with DS at any age. Neuronal densities were diminished from

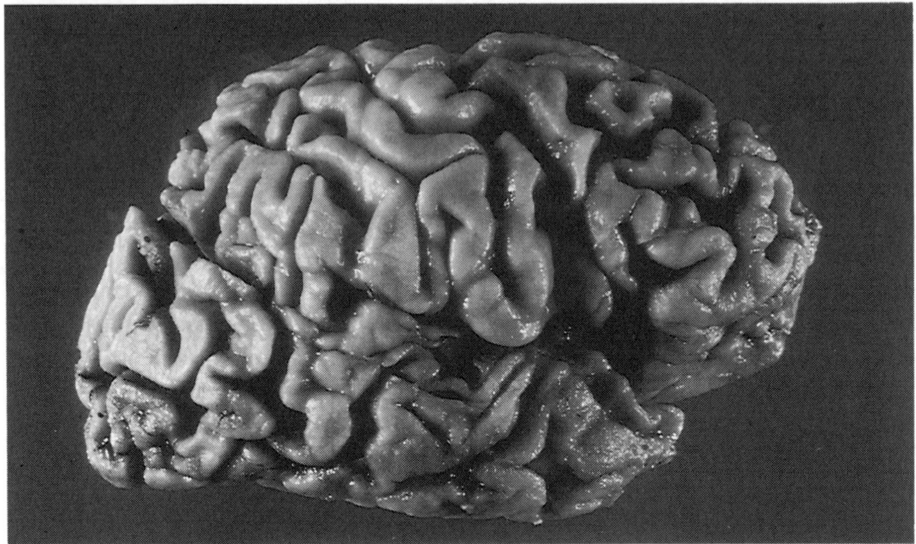

*Figure 1.2.* Postmortem study of a brain from a six-year-old DS female with bilateral severe narrowing of superior temporal gyrus, shortening of frontal and flattening of occipital lobes. She received early intervention, proper education, intensive speech therapy, and still expressive language was at 2 years and receptive at 5–6 year level.

10–50% in individuals with DS and this was noted already at birth (Wisniewski *et al.* 1986; Wisniewski 1990) (see Figure 1.3). The varying number of neurons reflected brain size. In individuals in whom there was greater reduction in the number of neurons, microcephaly was more common. In 20% of DS cases the number of neurons per square millimetre was within normal limits or borderline (10–20% decrease), while 30–50% decrease in neuronal densities was observed in 80% of these cases.

The distribution of neurons in the cortical layers in area 17 of individuals with DS showed decreased number of neurons, especially prominent in granular layers II and IV, compared with age-matched control subjects.

When synaptic densities and morphology were studied at the ultrastructural level, it was found that synaptic density is the greatest at around eight months of age and subsequently decreases, reaching adult values by nine years of age both in children with DS and in controls. Synaptic density in the visual cortex of individuals with DS is 10–29% lower than in control cases and this decrease is noted from birth (see Figure 1.4).

The morphology of synapses in DS reveals characteristic changes. Mean synaptic length was found to be changed during postnatal brain development. In non-DS control tissue, presynaptic and postsynaptic lengths increase throughout the examined ages. In this group the mean

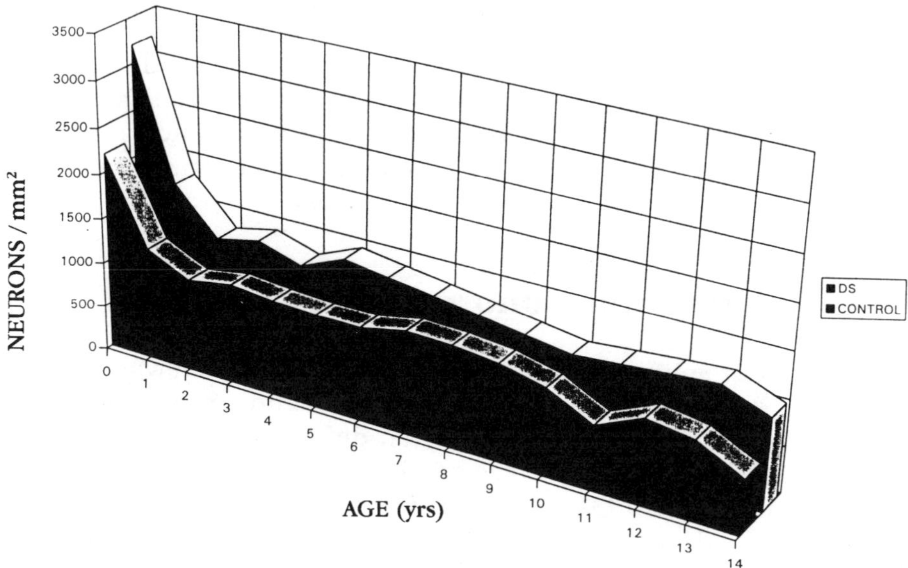


*Figure 1.3.* The mean of neuronal density in DS from birth to 14 years of age is lower than in the control cases. Similar abnormalities are found in the frontal and temporal lobes (not included).

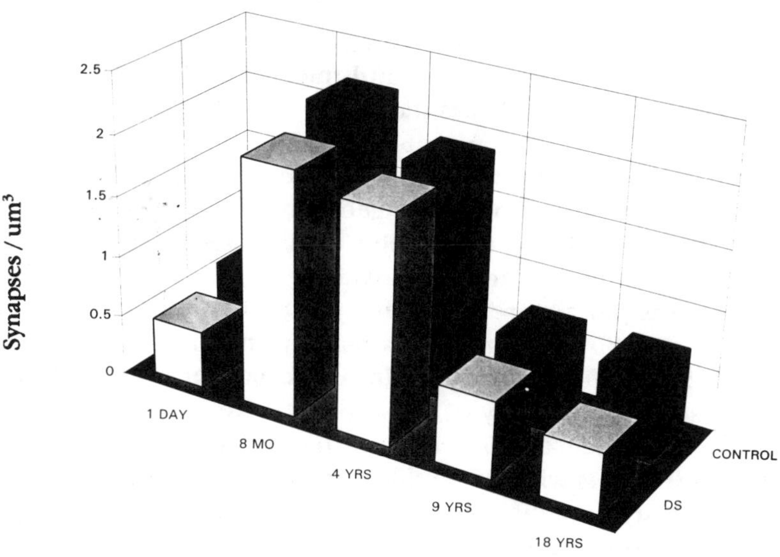


*Figure 1.4.* Synaptic density from day one to 18 years of age in DS is lower than the non-DS cases.

value in the newborn was 0.20 m, at 8 months 0.22 m, at 4 years 0.24 m, and at 9 and 18 years 0.28 m. In brains of individuals with DS, the average length of synapses was found to be diminished and to increase with age; for example, the length at one day was 0.18 m and at 18 years of age was 0.23 m. The average surface area per synaptic contact (see Figure 1.5), appears to be 20–35% less in the visual cortices of individuals with DS than in those of control individuals.

## 1.4 Hypothalamic Abnormalities

Recently, neuroendocrinological studies in some children with DS using tests for dopamine, clonidine stimulation and growth hormone-releasing factor (GH-RF) demonstrated deficiency of human growth hormone (hGH) secondary to hypothalamic dysfunction (Torrado *et al.* 1991; Castells *et al.* 1992, 1993; Wisniewski and Bobinski 1991). Good response to hGH therapy in children with DS could be demonstrated by increased somatic growth and head circumference (Annerén *et al.* 1986; Wisniewski *et al.* 1989; Torrado *et al.* 1991; Castells *et al.* 1992, 1993).

Immunohistochemical studies of the hypothalamus have revealed that the arcuate nucleus (ARC) and the ventromedial nucleus (VMN) are the sites of the highest concentrations of GH-RF (Bloch *et al.* 1983; Ling *et al.* 1984; Daikoku *et al.* 1986; Niimi *et al.* 1989; Ciofi *et al.* 1990). Because of the documented role of these hypothalamic nuclei in GH-RF production, we sought in our studies to examine the cytoarchitectonic organization of the hypothalamus in DS and control brains.

Brains of three individuals with DS secondary to trisomy-21 with severe mental and growth retardation and microcephaly and brains of three subjects without mental retardation were fixed in 10% phosphate-buffered formalin for periods of from 6–24 months. The ages of control subjects were 12, 20 and 29 years and of DS individuals, 12, 25 and 52 years. The brain weights of controls ranged between 1147 and 1180 g, whereas individuals with DS were between 790 and 990 g.

In the study (Wisniewski and Bobinski 1991), we found that the number of neurons per square millimetre in the hypothalamic nuclei (ARC and VMN) was 80% less in DS brains than in control brains (see Figure 1.5). This significant decrease in neuronal density suggests a decline in the secretory activity of these nuclei. We suppose that the decreased number of neurons observed in the hypothalamus and cerebral cortex of individuals with DS could be generalized to be present in the whole grey matter of the CNS, with some special topographical differences in certain brain areas, as was found in trisomy 16 mice (Sweeney *et al.* 1989). Hypothalamic studies must be performed in a larger number of cases to better define whether heterogeneity of pathological findings can be observed.

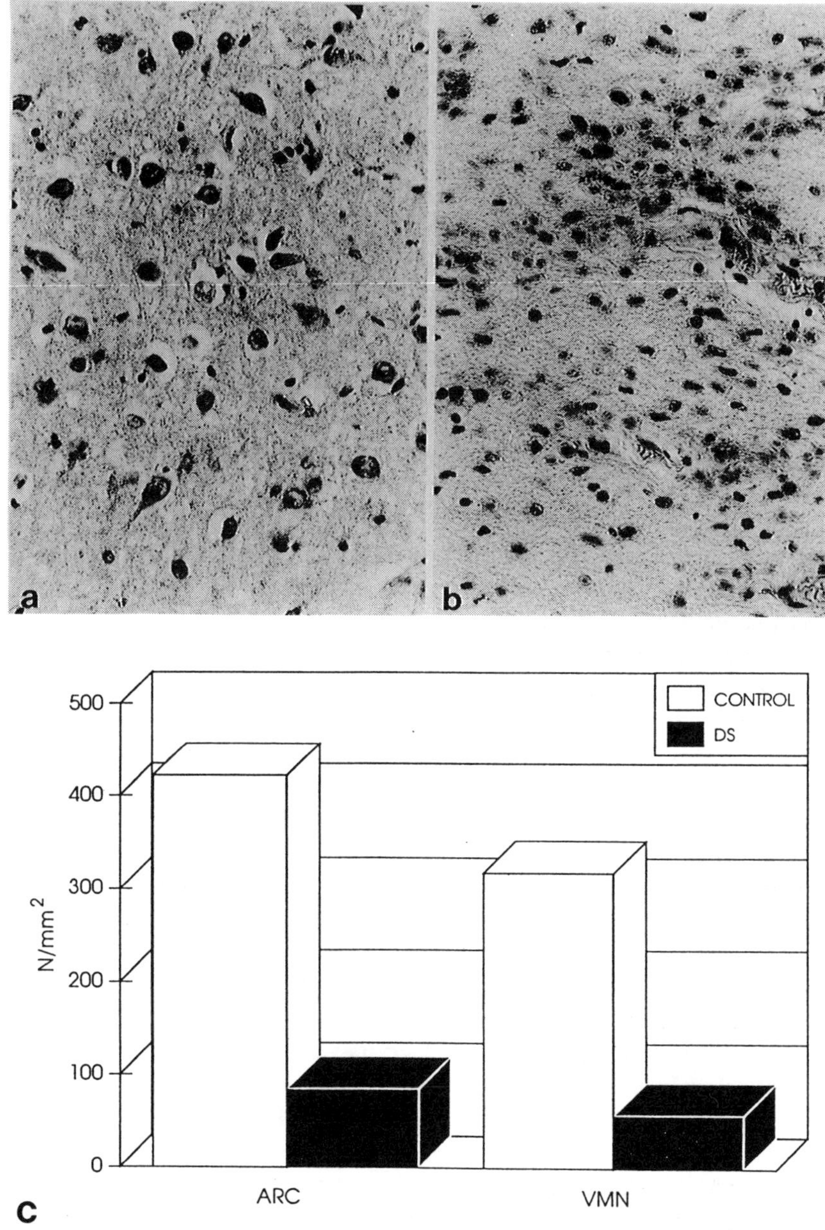


*Figure 1.5.* Neuronal density in arcuate nuclei (ARC) and ventromedial nuclei (VMN) in hypothalamic nuclei (5a., b. both at light microscopical level).

*5a.* Cells present in control hypothalamic ARC nucleus; x45.

*5b.* Cells present in DS hypothalamic ARC nucleus, x45. Please note the decreased number of neurons in DS hypothalamic ARC nucleus.

*5c.* The number of neurons per sq mm in ARC and VMN presented in bars – black bar: DS, white bar: control, (statistically analysed). Please note that the hypothalamic nuclei neurons were up to 80% less numerous in DS than in control cases (Wisniewski and Bobinski 1991).

## 1.5 Brain Abnormalities in Adult DS Subjects

Alzheimer's disease (AD) type of pathology was present in nearly all the brains we studied of individuals with DS who were 30 or 40 years of age or older at autopsy (Wisniewski *et al.* 1985b). The first, Aβ-positive, thioflavine S-negative plaques were found by us in DS subjects in the second decade of life. These deposits contained either moderate or low number of Aβ-positive fibrils as revealed by immunoelectron microscopy (Kida *et al.* 1995). Thioflavine-S-positive plaques, as well as classical and tau-1-positive neuritic plaques occur later and increases in their numerical density show a strong correlation with age (Wisniewski *et al.* 1995). Patients with DS frequently show higher density of senile plaques than patients with AD (Hof *et al.* 1995; Hyman *et al.* 1995). Neurofibrillary tangles appear later in DS subjects than β-amyloid deposits and their number gradually increases with age, until reaching, like amyloid deposits, a steady state beyond 50 years of age. The early vulnerability of entorhinal cortex and then of CA1/subiculum for neurofibrillary tangles is similar in DS subjects to that observed during normal ageing and AD (Hyman *et al.* 1995).

The inheritance of apolipoprotein E∑4 allele represents a risk factor for late-onset familial and sporadic AD (Saunders *et al.* 1993). In patients with AD, the∑4 allele frequency is significantly higher (0.5) than in the general population (0.12) (Strittmatter *et al.* 1993). In contrast to that, in patients with DS, the allelic frequency of the ∑4 allele is either similar to that in the general population (Saunders *et al.* 1993; Hardy *et al.* 1994) or even lower (Wisniewski *et al.* 1995). The distribution of apolipoprotein E within senile plaques in various brain regions of DS brain does not show significant differences as compared with AD brain (Kida *et al.* 1995). Moreover, patients with DS older than 50 years with the inheritance of the ∑4 allele show, like AD patients with ∑4 allele, higher amyloid burden than the subjects without allele ∑4 (Hyman *et al.* 1995). Thus, the apolipoprotein ∑4 genotype is an additional risk factor for developing higher levels of amyloid-β for DS subjects.

Clinico-pathological correlations suggested that dementia occurred in DS subjects many years later after the development of AD type of pathology in the brain tissue; usually beyond 50 years of age (Wisniewski *et al.* 1985a; 1985b; Lai and Williams 1989; Wisniewski *et al.* in press; see also Chapter 3 by Wisniewski and Silverman, in this volume). The duration of documented clinical manifestations of AD in DS cases is extending from 2.5 to 9.2 years before death (Wisniewski *et al.* 1985a).

Longitudinal prospective studies of adults with mild and moderate mental retardation who live in the community examined global changes in mental status and specific changes in auditory and visual memory over a period of seven years. Twenty-eight individuals with DS between 27 and 55 years of age were compared with 18 subjects without DS who were of similar IQ and age. The evaluation of mental status consisted of testing orientation to person, place and time, object naming, vasomotor coordination and concentration. Visual memory testing consisted of matching shapes, which were presented simultaneously and after delays of 0, 5 and 10 s on a computer-controlled screen. No changes were found in test scores between an initial testing and follow-up testing up to seven years later, indicating that ageing processes were not having a major impact in the cognitive functioning of these subjects (Devenny *et al.* 1992; Wisniewski *et al.* in press). Furthermore, there was no indication of any generalized decline in performance that would be suggestive of early symptoms of dementia among these subjects with DS. These longitudinal studies are still in progress and new data indicate that not only genetic, but environmental factors are of great importance in the development of AD in DS individuals.

## Acknowledgments

The authors wish to express their appreciation to Lawrence Black for bibliographical assistance and Jo-Ann Buttafuoco for secretarial assistance. Supported by Grant 9 PO1 AG 11531.

## References

Angevine Jr GB and Sidman RL (1961) Autoradiographic study of cell migration during histogenesis of cerebral cortex in the mouse. Nature 192: 766–8.

Annerén G, Sara VR, Hall K and Tuvemo T (1986) Growth and somatomedin responses to growth hormone in Down's syndrome. Archives of Disabilities in Childhood 6: 48–52.

Apert E (1914) Mongolism. Le Monde Médical 24: 201.

Benda CE (1969) Down's Anomaly (2nd Ed) New York: Grune and Stratton.

Benda CE (1971) Mongolism. In J Mencken (Ed) Pathology of the Nervous System 2: 1361–71. New York: McGraw-Hill.

Bloch B, Brazeau P, Ling N, Bohlen P, Esch F, Wehrenberg WB, Benoit R, Bloom F and Guillemin R (1983) Immunohistochemical detection of growth hormone-releasing factor in brain. Nature 301: 607–8.

Brooksbank BWL, Walker D, Balalzs R and Jorgensen OS (1989) Neuronal maturation in the fetal brain in Down's syndrome. Early Human Development 18: 237–46.

Castells S, Beaulieu I and Wisniewski KE (1993) Long-term effects of recombinant human growth hormone (rhGH) on children with Down's syndrome with short stature. In S Castells and KE Wisniewski (Eds) Growth hormone treatment in Down syndrome, pp. 163–82. New-York: Wiley.

Castells S, Torrado C, Bastian W and Wisniewski KE (1992) Growth hormone deficiency in Down's syndrome children. Journal of Intellectual Disability Research 36: 29-43.

Ciofi P, Tramu G and Bloch B (1990) Comparative immunohistochemical study of the distribution of neuropeptide Y, growth hormone-releasing factor and the carboxyterminus of precursor protein GHRF in the human hypothalamic infundibular area. Neuroendocrinology 51: 429–36.

Courchesne E (1988) Physioanatomical considerations in Down's syndrome. In L Nadel (Ed) The Psychobiology of Down Syndrome, pp.291-313. Cambridge MA: MIT Press.

Crome L, Cowie V and Slater E (1966) A statistical note on cerebellar and brain-stem weight in mongolism. Journal of Mental Deficiency Research 10: 69-72.

Crome L and Stern J (1972) Pathology of mental retardation. Baltimore MD: Williams and Wilkins.

Daikoku S, Kawano H, Noguchi M, Nakanishi J, Tokuzen M, Chihara K and Nagatsu I (1986) GRF neurons in the rat hypothalamus. Brain Research 399: 250–61.

Devenny DA, Hill AL, Patxot O, Silverman WP and Wisniewski KE (1992) Ageing in higher functioning adults with Down's syndrome: an interim report in a longitudinal study. Journal of Intellectual Disability Research 36: 241–50.

Friede RL (1989) Developmental neuropathology. Berlin: Springer.

Gans A (1925) Anatomische Beobachtungen bei der mongoloiden Idiotic. Nederlandse Tijdschrift Geneeskdunde 69: 922–5.

Garcia I, Martinou I, Tsujimoto Y and Martinou J-C (1992) Prevention of programmed cell death of sympathetic neurons by the bcl-2 proto-oncogene. Science 258: 302–4.

Golden JA and Hyman BT (1994) Development of the superior temporal neocortex is anomalous in trisomy 21. Journal of Neuoropathological Experimental Neurology 53: 513–20.

Gulotta F and Rehder H (1974) Chromosomal anomalies and central nervous system. Beiträge Pathologïe 152: 74–80.

Hardy J, Crook R, Perry Raghaven R and Roberts G (1994) Apo E genotype and Down's syndrome. (letter) Lancet 343: 979–80.

Haug H (1986) History of neuromorphometry. Journal of Neuroscience 18: 1–17.

Henderson DJ, Sherman LS, Loughna SC, Bennett PR and Moore GE (1994) Early embryonic failure associated with uniparental disomy for human chromosome 21. Human Molecular Genetics 3: 1373–6.

Hengartner MO, Ellis RE and Horvitz HR (1992) Caenorhabditis elegans gene ced-9 protects cells from programmed cell death. Nature 356: 494–9.

Hof PR, Bouras C, Perl DP, Sparks L, Mehta N and Morrison JH (1995) Archives of Neurology 52: 379–91.

Hyman BT, West HL, Rebeck GW, Lai F and Mann DMA (1995) Neuropathological changes in Down's syndrome hippocampal formation. Archives of Neurology 52: 373–8.

Jacob H (1956) Mongolismus. In O Lubarsch, F Henke and R Rossle (Eds) Erkrankungen des zentralen Nervensystems, Handbuch der speziellen pathologischen Anatomic u. Histologie. Bd. 13 Nervensystem, pp.82–98. Berlin: Springer.

Kemper TL (1988) Neuropathology of Down Syndrome. In L Nadel (Ed) The Psychobiology of Down's Syndrome, pp.269–89. Cambridge MA: MIT Press.

Kida E, Choi-Miura N-H and Wisniewski KE (1995) Deposition of apolipoproteins E and J in senile plaques is topographically determined in both Alzheimer's disease and Down's syndrome brain. Brain Research. 685: 211–216.

Korenberg JR, Chen X-N, Schipper R, Sun Z, Gonsky R, Gerwehr S, Carpenter N, Daumer C, Dignan P, Disteche C, Graham Jr JM, Hugdins L, McGillivray B, Miyazaki K, Ogasawara N, Park JP, Pagon R, Pueschel S, Sack G, Say B, Schuffenhauer S, Soukup S and Yamanaka T (1994) Down syndrome phenotypes. The consequences of chromosomal imbalance. Proceedings of the Natural Academy of Science 91: 4997–5001.

Lai F and Williams RS (1989) A prospective study of Alzheimer disease in Down syndrome. Archives of Neurology 46: 849–53.

Ling N, Esch F, Böhlen P, Brazeau P, Wehrenberg WB and Guillemin R (1984) Isolation, primary structure, and synthesis of human hypothalamic somatocrinin growth hormone-releasing factor. Proceedings of the Natural Academy of Science 81: 4302–6.

McKusick VA (1994) Mendelian inheritance in man. Baltimore MD: Johns Hopkins University Press.

Niimi M, Takahara J, Sato M and Kawanishi K (1989) Sites of origin of growth hormone-releasing factor-containing neurons projecting to the stalk-median eminence of the rat. Peptides 10: 605–8.

Palmer CGS, Cronk C, Pueschel SM, Wisniewski KE, Laxova R, Crocker AC and Pauli RM (1992) Head circumference of children with Down syndrome (0-36 months). American Journal of Medical Genetics 42: 61–7.

Petit TL, LeBoutillier JC, Alfano DP and Becker LE (1984) Synaptic development in the human fetus. A morphometric analysis of normal and Down's syndrome neocortex. Experimental Neurology 83: 13–23.

Price M, Lazzaro D, Pohl T, Mattei M-G, Rüther U, Olivo J-C, Duboule D and Di Lauro R (1992) Regional expression of the homeobox gene Nkx-2.2 in the developing mammalian forebrain. Neuron 8: 241–55.

Renucci A, Zappavigna V, Zàkàny J, Izpisùa-Belmonte J-C, Bürki K and Duboule D (1992) Comparison of mouse and human HOX-4 complexes defines conserved sequences involved in the regulation of HOX- 4.4. EMBO 11: 1459–68.

Roche AF (1966) The cranium in mongolism. Acta Neurologica Scandinavia 42: 62–78.

Rorke LB (1994) A perspective. The role of disordered genetic control of neurogenesis in the pathogenesis of migration disorders. Journal of Neuropathological Experimental Neurology 53: 105–17.

Ross MN, Galaburda AM and Kemper TL (1984) Down's syndrome, is there a decreased population of neurons? Neurology 34: 909–16.

Ruddle FH, Bartels JL, Bentley KL, Kappen C, Murtha MT and Pendleton JW (1994) Evolution of HOX Genes. Annual Review of Genetics 28: 423–42.

Saunders AM, Schmader K and Breitner JCS (1993) Apolipoprotein E ∑4 allele distributions in late-onset Alzheimer's disease and in other amyloid-forming diseases. Lancet 342: 710–11.

Schmidt-Sidor B, Wisniewski KE, Shepard TH and Sersen EA (1990) Brain growth in Down syndrome subjects 15 to 22 weeks of gestational age, and birth to 60 months. Clinical Neuropathology 9: 181–90.

Scott BS, Becker LE and Petit TL (1983) Neurobiology of Down's syndrome. Progress in Neurobiology 21: 199–237.

Scott BS, Petit TL, Becker LE and Edwards BAV (1982) Abnormal electric membrane properties of Down's syndrome DRG neurons in cell culture. Developmental Brain Research 2: 257–70.

Shawlot W and Behringer RR (1995) Requirement for Lim1 in head-organizer function. Nature 374: 425-30.

Sherman SL, Petersen MB, Freeman SB, Hersey J, Pettay D, Taft L, Frantzen M, Mikkelsen M and Hassold TJ (1994) Non-disjunction of chromosome 21 in maternal meiosis I: evidence for a maternal age-dependent mechanism involving reduced recombination. Human Molecular Genetics 3: 1529–35.

Sidman RL and Rakic P (1973) Neuronal migration with special reference to developing human brain. A review. Brain Research 62: 1–35.

Strittmatter WJ, Saunders AM, Schmechel D, Pericak-Vance M, Enghild J, Salvesen GS and Roses AD (1993) Apolipoprotein E: high-avidity binding to beta-amyloid and increased frequency of type 4 allele in late-onset familial Alzheimer disease. Proceedings of the Natural Academy of Science 90: 1977–81.

Stuart ET, Kioussi C and Gruss P (1993) Mammalian pax genes. Annual Review of Genetics 27: 219–36.

Sweeney JE, Höhmann CF, Oster-Granite ML and Coyle JT (1989) Neurogenesis of the basal forebrain in euploid and trisomy 16 mice an animal model for developmental disorders in Down syndrome. Neuroscience 31: 413–25.

Sylvester PE (1983) The hippocampus in Down's syndrome. Journal of Mental Deficiency Research 27: 227–36.

Takashima S, Becker LE, Armstrong DL and Chan F (1981) Abnormal neuronal development in the visual cortex of the human fetus and infant with Down's syndrome. A quantitative and qualitative Golgi study. Brain Research 225: 1–21.

Torrado C, Bastian W, Wisniewski KE and Castells S (1991) Treatment of children with Down syndrome and growth retardation with recombinant human growth hormone. Journal of Pediatrics 119: 478–83.

Wisniewski HM, Wegiel J and Popovitch ER (1994) Age-associated development of diffuse and thioflavin-S-positive plaques in Down syndrome. Developmental Brain Dysfunction 7: 330–339.

Wisniewski KE (1990) Down syndrome children often have brain with maturation delay, retardation of growth and cortical dysgenesis. American Journal of Medical Genetics 7: 274–81.

Wisniewski KE, Beaulieu I, Bobinski M, Lee MH and Castells S (1993) Microcephaly and neurological and neuropathological abnormalities in children with Down syndrome. In S Castells and KE Wisniewski (Eds) Growth hormone treatment in Down syndrome, pp.37–54. New York: Wiley.

Wisniewski KE and Bobinski M (1991) Hypothalamic abnormalities in Down syndrome. In CJ Epstein (Ed) The morphogenesis of Down syndrome, pp.153–67. New York: Wiley-Liss.

Wisniewski KE, Dalton AJ, McLachlan C, Wen GY and Wisniewski, HM (1985a) Alzheimer's disease in Down's syndrome clinicopathologic studies. Neurology 35: 957–61.

Wisniewski KE and Kida E (1995) Abnormal Neurogenesis and Synaptogenesis in Down Syndrome Brain. Developmental Brain Dysfunction 7: 289–301.

Wisniewski KE, Laure-Kamionowska M, Connell F and Wen GY (1986) Neuronal density and synaptogenesis in the postnatal stage of brain maturation in Down syndrome. In CJ Epstein (Ed) Neurobiology in Down syndrome, pp.29–44. New York: Raven Press.

Wisniewski KE, Laure-Kamionowska M and Wisniewski HM (1984) Evidence of arrest of neurogenesis and synaptogenesis in brains of patients with Down's syndrome. New England Journal of Medicine 311: 1187–8.

Wisniewski KE and Schmidt-Sidor B (1989) Postnatal delay of myelin formation in brains from Down syndrome infants and children. Clinical Neuropathology 2: 55–62.

Wisniewski KE, Torrado C and Castells S (1989) Treatment in growth hormone-deficient Down syndrome children with recombinant human growth hormone. Down's Syndrome for Professionals 12(4): 1–2.

Wisniewski KE, Wisniewski HM and Wen GY (1985b) Occurrence of neuropathological changes and dementia of Alzheimer's disease in Down's syndrome. Annal of Neurology 17: 278–82.

Wisniewski KE, Zimmerli E, Mlodzik B, Devenny DA and Wisniewski HM (in press) Aging and Alzheimer disease in Mild/Moderate Mentally Retarded Adults with Down Syndrome. In Collective, Congenital Disabilities and Aging, p.42. Milan: Italy: Omega Edizioni Via Cirenaica.

Wisniewski T, Morelli L, Wegiel J, Levy E, Wisniewski HM and Frangione B (1995) The influence over lipoprotein E isotopes on Alzheimer. Annal of Neurology 37: 136–8.

Yuan J and Horvitz HR (1990) The caenorhabditis elegans genes ced-3 and ced-4 act cell autonomously to cause programmed cell death. Developmental Biology 138: 33–41.

Zappavigna V, Renucci A, Izisùa-Belmonte JC, Urier G, Peschle C and Duboule D (1991) HOX4 genes encode transcription factors with potential auto- and cross-regulatory capacities. EMBO 10: 4177–87.

Zellweger H (1977) Down syndrome. In P Vinken and GW Bruyn (Eds) Handbook of Clinical Neurology 31: 367–469. Amsterdam: North Holland.

# 2

# Learning, Memory and Neural Function in Down's Syndrome

LYNN NADEL

## 2.1 Introduction

In this chapter I will discuss aspects of learning and memory in individuals with Down's syndrome (DS) in a framework provided by an analysis of the neural systems known to underlie various forms of learning and memory. It is now clear that there are multiple learning/memory systems (see Nadel 1992, 1994, for recent reviews), and in most clinical syndromes, such as Down's syndrome, Alzheimer's disease, Parkinsonism, and Huntington's chorea, impairments of learning and memory predominantly affect some, but rarely if ever all, of these forms of learning and memory. To the extent that one wishes to develop intervention strategies for infants and children with DS, it is essential to understand which learning and memory systems are disproportionately impaired, and which are not. It is also important to understand which, if any, of these impairments can be ameliorated and which not. This latter issue requires careful attention to the underlying neural correlates of the impairment, as well as to the cognitive structure of the various kinds of learning.

Accordingly, this chapter will begin with a discussion of the various kinds of learning and memory, briefly reviewing some of the data that have demonstrated the existence and nature of these multiple systems. It will continue with a review of what is known about the neural impairments associated with DS, and how these might impact the various types of learning and memory discussed in the opening section. Following this, it will review current knowledge about learning and memory in individuals with DS, from a wide range of learning situations. The final section will draw some conclusions about the range of effects one sees in learning/memory performance in individuals with DS, the kinds of information that we still lack and sorely need if we are to fully understand this syndrome's impact on learning and memory, and what we can now assume as a basis for the development of intervention methods.

## 2.2 The Nature of Learning and Memory

In recent years it has become clear that learning and memory functions cannot be characterized in a singular fashion, either in terms of their behavioural and cognitive properties, or in terms of the neural systems upon which they rest. Initially in work with animals (Nadel and O'Keefe 1974; O'Keefe and Nadel 1978) and subsequently in work with humans (Cohen and Squire 1980), it has been shown that there are multiple learning and memory systems with distinct properties and neural bases. These distinctions are critically important in understanding the precise nature of various clinical syndromes such as amnesia, Alzheimer's disease, and, I will argue here, Down's syndrome. Understanding the nature and specific roles of multiple memory systems is relevant to the proper characterization of DS because the neural dysfunctions observed in this (and most other syndromes) are not spread evenly throughout the brain: rather, they affect some parts of the brain more than others. To the extent that different brain regions are essential for quite different forms of learning and memory, it is critical to determine what kinds of learning and memory exist, what brain regions are responsible for each type, and what brain regions are particularly compromised in DS. Only when we have answers to all these questions will we be able to state with some assurance just what aspects of learning and memory are especially at risk in this syndrome. Such information is particularly important in deciding what sorts of educational programmes to emphasize in this, and other developmental, syndromes. A recent review of the efficacy of early intervention programmes notes that there has been scant application of knowledge about the specific learning abilities and disabilities of DS individuals to the development of these programmes (Gibson and Harris 1988). Wishart (1993) refused to accept the pessimistic conclusion that there is a low and immutable barrier to the advancement of children with DS, noting that in these children the 'developmental rate may not be responding to current educational input because that input is in some way inappropriate in its structure, in its timing, or at an even more basic level, in its theoretical underpinnings' (p.391).

### 2.2.1 Types of learning and memory

Some time ago O'Keefe and I (1978) proposed that a particular part of the brain, the *hippocampus*, was involved in a highly specific form of learning and memory that we called 'cognitive mapping'. We contrasted the kind of learning carried out by this brain region (and its collaborating neighbours) with other forms of learning that did not have the same map-like qualities. Table 2.1 indicates the key features of the two main classes of learning that we postulated, which we called 'locale' and 'taxon' learning. The names locale and taxon were chosen to reflect central distinguishing features of these two types of learning. Locale learning always incorporates information about where objects and events are located; taxon learning, by contrast, does not incorporate such contextual information, focusing instead on the conceptual and categorical information obtained through experiences in the environment. As Table 2.1 shows, these two types of learning differ in many important respects. Locale learning is assumed to be rapid, one-trial, easily changed, flexible in use, related to the context in which it is obtained (e.g., episodic), and acquired without regard to standard biological motivations such as food, water and safety. Taxon learning, on the other hand, is assumed, generally, to be relatively slow, incremental, persistent and changed only with difficulty, inflexible in use, not related to the context in which it is obtained, and typically acquired in relation to the action of biological rewards.

Table 2.1 Two types of learning and their properties

| | *Locale Learning* | *Taxon Learning* |
|---|---|---|
| Speed of learning | Rapid, One-trial | Slow, Incremental |
| Persistence | Easily changed | Highly persistent |
| Flexibility | High | Low |
| Contextual links | Linked to context | Unlinked to context |
| Motivation | Curiosity | Biological reward |
| Representation | Map-like/Relational | Categorical |

Locale and taxon learning systems are distinguished also by the nature of the representations they establish i.e., the way in which they 'store' acquired information. Within the locale system information is stored in a map-like representation (hence the use of the term 'cognitive map' to describe the hippocampus) such that all parts of an acquired memory stand in some relation to all other parts. In this way, one part of an episode memory can serve as a retrieval cue for another part. Further, this form of relational storage permits inferences between and among parts of the memory that might never have occurred together. For example, we can figure out the relations between two parts of a city even though we have never gone from one to the other because they are both part of a larger relational structure. In the same vein, we can use this structure to generate new 'paths' from one place to another, whether we are talking about real places in the environment or just figurative places in some learned representation. The term 'map' is used here not to imply that there is a literal map in the brain, but rather that the underlying neural system, in this case in the hippocampus, functions as though it had the properties of maps as just described.

In contrast, within the taxon systems information is stored by virtue of categorical relations, with links between categories established through pairwise associations. We have likened this form of representation to a 'route' to contrast it with the web-like nature of maps. These route-like representations do not have the kind of flexibility, nor do they permit the sort of inferences associated with maps. Hence, the kind of learning, and what can be done with the information acquired, varies in important ways between the locale and taxon systems.

We argued that these two kinds of learning were subserved by different regions in the brain, and indeed, that the properties that distinguish them derive in large measure from the underlying computational structure of the neural systems involved. As noted above, we supposed that locale learning was dependent upon the hippocampus and neighbouring structures in the medial temporal lobe of the brain. Taxon learning was supposed to be dependent upon other parts of the cerebral cortex, basal ganglia and various other subcortical structures. We pointed out that there were many types of taxon learning and that different types were likely to be subserved by different brain regions. Taxon learning includes not only the category learning noted above, but also the learning of skills, habits and procedures, which can be viewed as motor concepts.

Of course, these two separate learning systems are not independent from one another. We postulated that information flowed into the hippocampal learning system through the taxon systems, and that using the map-like information in the hippocampus required activation of appropriate information in these other brain areas. We have further speculated that the rapidly-formed memories in the hippocampal system contribute to the consolidation of memories in other brain regions (Squire *et al.* 1984; McClelland *et al.* 1992), and that in the absence of the hippocampus there might be problems with this consolidation process. I will return to this important point later.

More recent work by numerous other investigators in a range of species has largely confirmed the notion that there are essentially two types of learning systems, and that these are to be distinguished along the lines of the properties spelled out in Table 2.1 (Mishkin *et al.* 1984; Sutherland and Rudy 1989; Squire 1992; Cohen and Eichenbaum 1993; Schacter and Tulving 1994; Nadel 1992, 1994). This emerging synthesis on the nature of multiple learning and memory systems does not mean that there is complete agreement on all the details, of course, but there is sufficient agreement to permit those with clinical interests in syndromes in which there are learning/memory difficulties to make certain predictions about the nature of those problems if they can be based on knowledge of the underlying neural defects. There is considerable evidence that in a variety of syndromes, impairments in memory reflect these distinctions among types of memory.

In so far as one can be certain of the neural concomitants of DS and be confident about the kinds of learning and memory the affected neural regions are central to, one ought to be able to make specific predictions about the learning and memory abilities and disabilities of individuals with DS. This is, to be sure, a very simplistic way to approach the matter. For although every individual with DS who is trisomic for chromosome 21 starts from the same point, the range of abilities in this population, and the range of neural dysfunctions, is quite staggering. This range, paradoxically, holds out great hope, because if some individuals can attain great things, then this must, in a theoretical sense at least, be possible for all. (For further discussion of this point, see Rondal 1994, and Chapter 7 of this volume.)

## 2.3 Neural Sequellae of Down's Syndrome

What then do we currently know of the precise neural sequellae of DS? This turns out to be a more difficult question to answer than one might imagine at first glance, because we are dealing with a moving target. Data from a wide range of studies indicate that at birth there is apparently little to differentiate the brains of normal and DS individuals. Yet, both postmortem studies and various, more recent, non-invasive neuroimaging studies, have demonstrated rather clear differences between these two groups as early as six months of age. Where do these differences come from, and what do they amount to?

An immediately obvious difference is that the brains of individuals with DS are typically smaller than those of age-matched controls, at least after six months of age. However, one possibility that has been given insufficient attention in the past, but which must be looked at more carefully, is that this difference is merely a consequence of the fact that DS individuals are smaller overall. That is, the differences in brain size could be merely a matter of *allometry*. This possibility, taken in conjunction with the fact that there is no clear relation between brain size and 'intelligence' in any event, suggests that the mental retardation observed in DS is likely to result from something other than gross differences in brain size.

It is not simply that the brains of DS individuals are smaller overall, but that there are certain brain areas that are disproportionately affected, while others are affected quite minimally. This differential impact is not predicted by allometry, and must be considered very carefully in any attempt to draw conclusions from the study of neuropathology. Before discussing these specific problems there is another factor that must be taken into account: the probability that brain development is influenced by experience in highly important ways. If this is true, and there are increasing reasons from a range of basic neurobiological studies to believe that it is, then the study of the brains of individuals with DS who have recently come to postmortem evaluation might be quite misleading. Most of these individuals did not benefit from the kinds of early stimulation regimes that are now available and indeed prevalent, and that might have a direct impact on brain development. This is at present a highly speculative but very important area; as noted above, such brain plasticity is one of the best hopes for bringing about significant improvements in the development of individuals with DS. At this time we do not know, from a theoretical or empirical perspective, the extent to which experience can cause changes in normal brain development. We do not know whether normal possibilities for brain plasticity exist in individuals with DS. We do not know the extent to which changes in brain development that are promoted by specific stimulation regimes can translate into meaningful behavioural and cognitive improvements. We do not know which kinds of changes would be beneficial and which not. Obviously, there is a great deal we do not know in this area, and very little that we can be certain of, except that further research on these issues is of the utmost importance. While one does not wish to raise false hopes, it is important to stress that we now know the brain to be much more malleable than was previously thought.

With these caveats registered, what can we say about nervous system function in DS? At the outset, it is critical to separate the question, and our answers, into at least three developmental stages. First, it is important to know what the nervous system is like at or before birth, to get a sense of the starting point. Second, we need to know what the nervous system is like as the individual with DS develops through childhood, adolescent and into adult life. Third, we need to know what happens in the nervous system as the individual with DS reaches old age, which, as has now become clear, happens earlier in the DS population than in the normal population. Information about each of these stages is available, and will be briefly reviewed in what follows. This information comes from three primary sources: ***neuroanatomical studies*** of brains from individuals with DS who died at various ages, ***neurophysiological studies*** of the dynamic properties of the brains of individuals with DS at various ages, and ***neuroimaging studies*** of the metabolic activity of the brains of individuals with DS, typically in adulthood. Let us consider each of these briefly in turn. Further details on much of this can be found in the contributions of K. Wisniewski and H. Wisniewski in Chapters 1 and 3.

### 2.3.1 Early development

A wide range of studies points to the conclusion already noted, that the brain of an individual with DS at or shortly before birth is in many respects indistinguishable from the brain of a normal individual (Brooksbank *et al.* 1989; Wisniewski and Schmidt-Sidor 1989; Schmidt-Sidor *et al.* 1990; Florez *et al.* 1990; Bar-Peled *et al.* 1991; Pazos *et al.* 1994). Normal values have been reported for brain and skull shape, brain weight, proportion of specific cerebral lobes, size of cerebellum and brain stem, and the emergence of most neurotransmitter systems. The fact that relative normalcy exists at birth is potentially of the greatest significance, since it seems to create the opportunity to do something about the not-yet-created differences that quite clearly do emerge during the period right after birth.

There is evidence, however, that some changes begin to emerge as early as 22 weeks gestational age (Schmidt-Sidor *et al.* 1990), and it is clear that by the age of six months a number of important differences are already obvious. Some of these differences are expressed in terms of the proportion of individuals with DS who show abnormal values, rather than in terms of a uniform abnormality in all instances. This too is of importance, as it highlights the variability in this population, a variability that attests to the critical role of environmental (epigenetic) factors in determining the phenotype in Down's syndrome, given the uniform genotypic feature of trisomy 21[1]. One quite noticeable difference concerns a postnatal delay in myelination, global at first but then manifested primarily in nerve tracts that are myelinated especially late in development, such as the fibres linking the frontal and temporal lobes; this delay is observed in about 25% of infants with DS between the ages of two months and six years. While not underestimating the impact of this myelination delay, it is certainly worth noting that in all cases myelination is within normal range at birth, while in 75% of the cases it is within normal range throughout early development.

Neuropathological differences after three to five months of age include a shortening of the fronto-occipital length of the brain that appears to result from a reduction in growth of the frontal lobes, a narrowing of the superior temporal gyrus (observed in about 35% of cases), a diminished size of the brain stem and cerebellum (observed in most cases) and a significant reduction (20–50%) in the number of cortical granular neurons (see Benda 1971; Crome *et al.* 1966; Blackwood and Corsellis 1976). There is some indication in the data of a relation between the occurrence of neuropathological abnormalities and other problems in DS, such as congenital heart disease. Notwithstanding these differences, however, the overall picture in infancy is one of relative normalcy, although individuals with DS tend to fall towards the bottom of the normal range (or outside it) in most measures.

Investigations of neural function, as opposed to structure, in early infancy suggest some abnormalities: in particular there is evidence of either delayed or aberrant auditory system development (Jiang *et al.* 1990) that might contribute to the widespread hearing disorders observed in Down's syndrome. Obviously, such a disorder, if organic, could be related to many of the subsequent difficulties seen in the learning of language. There is also evidence of a more widespread abnormality in EEG coherence that seems to reflect a generally impoverished dendritic environment. This difference, like many of the others, emerges only sometime after birth (McAlaster 1992). It appears that this effect is predominant in posterior, rather than anterior, brain regions, and in the left, more than the right, hemisphere.

### 2.3.2 Childhood, adolescence and early adulthood

The evidence of neuropathological sequellae in Down's syndrome is more extensive for the middle stage of life. Data from both postmortem studies and from studies of brain function in select populations, indicates that the changes beginning to emerge early in life become more prominent and prevalent by early adolescence. Thus, Becker *et al.* (1986) showed that dendritic arborizations in visual cortex of individuals with DS were paradoxically greater than normal early in infancy, but then considerably less than normal by the age of two years. They speculate that the initial overabundance might result from a compensatory response to the absence of adequate synapse formation, but the basic point remains that by early childhood there is an impoverishment in neocortex. This increasing deficit in neocortical microstructure has been confirmed by Wisniewski; and as we have already observed, myelination is delayed in a significant number of children with DS (Wisniewski and Schmidt-Sidor 1989).

There have been relatively few studies of brain function in adolescents and young adults with DS, and the existing data are somewhat equivocal. Devinsky *et al.* (1990) reported relatively normal EEG alpha activity in young adults (< 40 years of age), while Shapiro *et al.* (1992) reported relatively normal brain metabolism in a similar group, using positron emission tomography (PET) measures of glucose uptake and regional blood flow. They did report some disruption of normal neuronal interactions between the frontal and parietal lobes, possibly including the language area of Broca. Overall, they concluded that in younger subjects with DS there is not generally cerebral atrophy beyond what would be predicted by the smaller cranial vault and stature of these subjects. On the other hand, in those cases where dementia can be observed in younger subjects, there are clear signs of abnormal cerebral atrophy and metabolic deficiencies. Enlargement of the ventricles is a standard sign in these cases. In an earlier study looking at glucose uptake these investigators found abnormal interactions between the thalamus and neocortex, in particular the temporal and occipital lobes, speculating that there might be a problem with 'directed attention' as a result (Horwitz *et al.* 1990). A study of EEG coherence (McAlaster 1992) reported abnormal development of EEG profiles in subjects with DS, with a particular emphasis again on the posterior cortical regions.

A recent PET study of seven young adults with DS (mean age 28 years) without dementia (Haier *et al.* 1995) confirmed previous findings that overall cortical glucose metabolic rate is higher in subjects with DS (and in other mentally retarded subjects) than in normal controls. This seemingly paradoxical increase is typically interpreted as a sign of 'inefficiency'[2]. When one looks at specific areas more closely, there are decreases in metabolic rate in medial frontal and medial temporal lobes in the DS subjects, and some evidence of dysfunction in the basal ganglia.

Overall, the evidence from the study of subjects in mid-life is still inconclusive. While there are clear problems in some cases, with some evidence for localized neuropathology, the general picture is quite diffuse. This, however, is not the case when one looks at studies focused on somewhat older subjects.

### 2.3.3 Late adulthood: the emergence of the signs of Alzheimer's disease

For some years it has been clear that neuropathology resembling that seen in Alzheimer's disease (AD) is prevalent in individuals with DS after the age of about 35 years. A large number of studies has concentrated on this issue, documenting the ways in which the neuropathology seen in Down's syndrome is similar to, or different from, that seen in Alzheimer's disease. A very important fact emerging from the past five years of careful study, is that while virtually 100% of individuals with DS show neuropathology similar to that associated with AD, less than 50% show the dementia invariably seen with AD. This uncoupling of the neuropathology from the dementia has, of course, occasioned considerable interest, with an initial emphasis on attempts to determine if there might be subtle differences between the cases of DS and AD that could explain the dissociation observed in DS but not in AD. It has not been possible to point to any such difference that could be said, with confidence, to account for this fact (Cork 1990). Recently, H. Wisniewski (see Chapter 3) has shown that there is a critical difference between DS and AD with regard to the nature of the amyloid deposits found in the plaques characteristic of the neuropathology common in these two syndromes. Dementia is only observed when insoluble amyloid, which causes the formation of fibrous tangles, is present. This type of amyloid is rarely seen in DS until after 50 years of age, regardless of the extent of gross neuropathology.

Two recent papers provide an up-to-date view on the neuropathology observed in adults with DS (Kesslak *et al.* 1994; Raz *et al.* in press). The first study looked at 13 adults with DS, using magnetic resonance imaging (MRI) to assess the size of various brain regions. Two additional subjects with clinically diagnosed dementia were also studied. The main findings in the group without dementia were a decrease in the size of the hippocampus and neocortex, and a paradoxical increase in the size of the parahippocampal gyrus. No significant differences were observed in the superior temporal lobe, the middle and inferior temporal lobes, the lateral ventricles, or cortical or subcortical areas. In these DS subjects there were only two significant age-related changes: with ageing, ventricle size increased and hippocampal size decreased. In the two subjects with dementia, there was considerable brain atrophy and an enlargement of the ventricles; in general a picture similar to that observed in Alzheimer's disease, but absent in the subjects with DS who were not clinically demented, even those as old as 51 years of age.

The second study looked at 25 adults, 13 with DS, also using MRI. Most critically, their results were adjusted for body size, so they took into account differences resulting simply from allometry. The authors found that a number of brain regions were smaller in the DS subjects, including the hippocampal formation, the mammillary bodies, and parts of the cerebellum and cerebral hemispheres. They also replicated the increase in size of the parahippocampal gyrus observed by Kesslak *et al.* (1994), and found that it was highly correlated with the cognitive defect in their subjects. There was some shrinkage of other brain regions, including the dorsolateral prefrontal cortex, the anterior cingulate cortex, the pericalcarine cortex, the inferior temporal and parietal cortex, and the parietal white matter. No differences at all were observed in orbitofrontal cortex, pre- and post-central gyri, and the basal ganglia.

These observed changes confirm earlier reports of decreased volume of cerebellum (Jernigan and Bellugi 1990; Weis 1991), and of decreased dendritic spines and volume in the hippocampus (Ferrer and Gullotta 1990). There have also been reports of neuropathology in the amygdala (Mann and Esiri 1989; Murphy *et al.* 1992), in particular in those subregions most closely associated with the hippocampus (Murphy and Ellis 1991).

The earliest neuropathological changes with ageing in DS seem to appear in parts of the hippocampal formation, especially the entorhinal cortex, but also involving the dentate gyrus, CA1 and the subiculum (Mann and Esiri 1989; Hyman 1992). There is extensive cell loss in the locus coeruleus (Mann *et al.* 1990), a brainstem nucleus that projects to the hippocampal formation; this was most noticeable in cases of severe dementia.

In summary, there are widespread signs of neuropathology in older subjects with DS, but there is a selectivity nonetheless, in terms of where signs are seen first, and where they are most prominent. In this regard, changes in hippocampal formation (Ball and Nuttal 1981; Sylvester 1983; Ball *et al.* 1986), temporal lobe in general (Deb *et al.* 1992; Spargo *et al.* 1992) and cerebellum (Cole *et al.* 1993) stand out.

Overall, study of neuropathology in early and later life points to certain regions of the cortex, including most prominently the temporal lobe[3] and the hippocampal formation (Wisniewski *et al.* 1986), and to the cerebellum[4]. In analysing learning and memory difficulties, then, we should be particularly alert to those kinds of changes that might reflect particular problems with these neural systems.

## 2.4 Learning and Memory in Individuals with Down's Syndrome

In considering the learning and memory abilities of individuals with DS the two major concerns already discussed must be taken into account: first, learning and memory must be considered as involving a number of separate systems; and second, attention must be paid to the abilities of individuals at various stages of life. It is clear from a review of existing studies that some brain systems are affected more than others, and that these brain systems are responsible for only some, but not all, kinds of learning. I would like to focus on one of the conclusions from this review – that parts of the medial temporal lobe, in particular the hippocampus, seem disproportionately affected in DS. The evidence for this is now quite clear in older subjects, if only suggestive in younger subjects. As noted earlier, the hippocampal system is involved in spatial cognition in particular, flexible learning in general, and the normal consolidation of what has already been learned. It is known that this system is not crucial for much learning about categories and concepts, nor is it necessary for skill learning. Unfortunately, we do not have as clear a picture of the precise functions of the cerebellum, another brain region prominently affected in subjects with DS. There is some evidence to suggest that it is involved in motor skills, and other indications that it might be critical in the acquisition of conditioned responses, for example the so-called *nictitating membrane* response. We will see below that there is some evidence that this form of conditioning is indeed impaired in older subjects with DS.

Before attributing particular problems with learning and memory to specific neuropathologies, we must take into account difficulties that individuals with DS might have in sensory and perceptual function that could contribute to or account for these learning problems. As we have already noted, there are indications of an organic basis for hearing difficulties that could certainly compromise language learning (Marcell and Cohen 1992). There is, in addition, evidence of a defect in visual acuity (Courage *et al.* 1994) that could contribute to problems with learning in situations where visual information is critical. Such indications suggest that early stimulation programmes must be sensitive to sensory and perceptual function, in the hope of maximizing capacities in these areas that might otherwise be suboptimal, thereby imposing a limit on the learning process. There are also difficulties on the motor side that must be taken into account in evaluating learning ability (Henderson 1985).

Once these more peripheral difficulties have been considered, what evidence do we have of further difficulties in learning and memory, and how might these relate to underlying neural dysfunction?

### 2.4.1 Early learning

In general, infants with DS show relatively normal abilities in learning and memory (but see Hepper and Shahidullah 1992, for a report of impaired habituation in two fetuses with DS). It is essential to understand, however, that this does not mean that either they, or indeed normally-developing infants, have the full adult range of learning and memory abilities at birth. In fact, this is not the case, since some parts of the brain mature postnatally, and the forms of learning and memory dependent on them are not available until some time after birth. The medial temporal lobe, and particularly the hippocampus, as well as parts of the cerebellum, are included in this category. The fact that these late-developing structures are apparently particularly at risk in Down's syndrome is probably of considerable importance (Nadel 1986). Although there is insufficient evidence to be certain about the exact ages, there is little doubt that in humans, as in most other animals, the hippocampus is not fully functional until many months after birth, and perhaps as long as 16–18 months (Nadel and Zola-Morgan 1984; Nadel and Willner 1989). This means that the kinds of learning and memory that are dependent upon this system are not available to infants.

In an early series of studies, Ohr and Fagen (1991, 1993) looked at the ability of infants to acquire behaviours based on learning about the *contingencies* between their own movements (leg-kicking) and reinforcement. They reported that three-month-old infants with DS were entirely normal at this task, including initial learning, acquisition speed, and retention. In a later report, (Ohr and Fagen 1994), they showed that nine-month-old infants with DS were impaired, as a group, in learning about the contingency between arm movements and reinforcement. However, they noted that *some* infants with DS were able to learn. They concluded that, after six months, there is a relative decline in conditionability in infants with DS compared with normally developing infants. This is in agreement with the general picture emerging from studies of brain maturation, which also show relative normalcy at birth but increasing abnormality after six months.

Mangan (1992) tested control infants and infants with DS on a variety of spatial tasks, one of which, a place-learning task, was designed especially to assess the state of function of the hippocampal system. It is known that this place-learning task does not emerge in normal development until about 18 months of age, which matches current estimates of when the hippocampus itself becomes functional (Mangan and Nadel 1990). Two other spatial tasks were utilized, one involving response-learning, where the child had to make a consistent body-turn, and the other involving cue-learning, where the child had to approach a specific cue. In all three tasks the child was searching for a toy hidden in a hole. After learning, the infants were removed from the apparatus for a delay interval, then were given a 'memory' test. Mangan tested children at the age of 16–20 months on the response and cue tasks and at the age of 26–30 months on the place task. He found that children with DS were somewhat impaired in the learning of all three tasks, although they did manage to learn them all. On the critical memory probes, children with DS performed similarly to the normal children on the response and cue tasks but were severely impaired on the place task. This pattern of results is consistent with diffuse, but mild, neuropathology combined with much more extensive pathology localized to the hippocampus.

In another study of spatial abilities, Uecker, Obrzut and Nadel (1994) showed that children with DS had difficulties in a task requiring the mental rotation of a stick-figure, when compared with another group of learning disabled children. Although capable of representing the stimulus in imagery, the children with DS were impaired at the spatial–transformational task of rotating that image. How, if at all, this relates to the spatial defect observed in place learning remains to be determined.

A great deal of work on learning within the language domain has been carried out in children with DS (see Rondal, Chapter 7; Buckley, Chapter 8). There is little question that difficulties in the acquisition of language can be quite severe, but there are also cases where language capacity is within normal range, or even at the upper end of that range. While it is hard to pinpoint the precise defect at the root of the typical language problem, there is little to suggest that the difficulty is primarily one of learning or memory. Infants with DS show many of the normal features of pre-language behaviour, including babbling and imitation, although there are some subtle but possibly important differences between DS and normally-developing infants in this regard (Lynch *et al.* in press). Vocalization appears to be under contingent control in infants with DS (Poulson 1988), and their ability to acquire words seems normal as well, although slow (Hopmann and Nothnagle 1994). As the focus of this chapter is on learning and memory, it will not consider the acquisition of language in any further detail.

In a series of longitudinal studies, Wishart (1993; see Chapter 6) has carefully examined the performance of children with DS in contingency detection tasks, on standard intelligence tests, and in terms of the development of the *object concept*. I will only briefly summarize this work here; in Chapter 6 Wishart provides a full description. Contingency learning was studied in a situation in which infants could produce rotation of a brightly coloured mobile by a kick that would break a light beam. Normally-developing infants can learn the contingency by two months of age, which involves kicking at a rate of 1.5 × baseline (taken as the kicking rate during a period when the contingency was not in effect). Children with DS were impaired in acquiring this task, but beyond that, the differences in how they performed are quite revealing. Wishart utilized several different reward schedules which varied in the extent to which subjects received 'free' (non-contingent) rewards. Counterintuitively, such rewards diminished the extent to which children with DS participated in controlling the rotation of the mobile themselves. Although these children maintained an interest in the task well beyond the age at which normally-developing children ceased, this interest was satisfied by passive acceptance of free rewards as readily as by active participation in gaining the rewards. This apparently fundamental difference between learning styles could be of the utmost importance in developing effective intervention programmes for the children with DS.

In the object concept situation, children with DS seemed to acquire the basic concept at more or less the same time as normally-developing infants. However, a different kind of problem emerged in this task: instability of acquisition. Although the typical subject with DS solved various levels of the tasks used to assess the object concept at ages not very far from the norm, performance after that could be highly variable and apparently beset by motivational difficulties. Once again, these problems, if representative of the learning style of children with DS, are extremely important in thinking about effective intervention. The results of Wishart's studies using standard intelligence test batteries suggest that they are indeed representative. Test–retest reliability was very low because successes gained in one test might not appear upon retest, as soon as two weeks later. New skills show up, only to disappear shortly thereafter.

The motivational difficulties and developmental instabilities observed in Wishart's work strongly suggest that young children with DS are not merely delayed in mental development, but actually follow a somewhat different path. As Wishart (1993) points out, this view 'has the substantial merit of being consistent with data from the neurosciences showing DS to be associated with fundamental differences in the morphology and functioning of the brain' (p. 392).

To summarize the situation in infants and children: there is evidence of relatively normal learning of certain types, especially in the youngest subjects. There is also evidence for some highly specific learning deficits, which typically emerge only some months or even years after birth. In the latter category there is evidence consistent with a specific problem in the hippocampal formation spatial cognitive system. There is also evidence that early development in DS is not only quantitatively slow, but is also qualitatively different.

The learning and memory problems that begin to emerge in late infancy become considerably more noticeable as the infant grows to childhood and adolescence. Most of our knowledge for this period comes from the learning of language, but there is some information available about other kinds of learning and memory. The major point to be stressed from these data has less to do with the inability of children with DS to acquire words, or linguistic constructions, or other non-verbal material, and more to do with their inability to 'stabilize' the information that they do manage to acquire. Wishart (1993) and Fowler (1988) stress this point, which might reflect, among other factors, impairments in the consolidation function earlier attributed to the hippocampal system.

### 2.4.2 Adulthood and ageing

A great deal of recent research has focused on the deterioration of learning, memory and other cognitive capacities as individuals with DS reach the age of 35 or older. As noted earlier, at this age one can be reasonably certain that at least some signs of neuropathology will be present in the brain of individuals with DS. The relation between this pathology and the onset of dementia and eventually Alzheimer's disease, is being actively studied at present. Here more than anywhere else, the notion that we are studying a 'moving target' is relevant. As more individuals with DS reach older ages in relatively good health, and as a higher proportion of these individuals will have enjoyed the benefits of early intervention programmes, and increased expectations, the picture of Down's syndrome capabilities might change. Given our earlier comments about brain plasticity, it is even possible that the certainty of neuropathology will change. There is a clear need to find ways to determine, prospectively if possible, those ageing subjects with Down's syndrome who are most at risk for the development of the clinical signs of AD. In this regard, recent work on emotional functioning in Down's syndrome, and changes with ageing, could be helpful (Nelson *et al.* in press).

One sign of this possibility is emerging in the work of Wisniewski's group (see Chapters 1 and 3); their current work on visual and auditory memory in high-functioning subjects between 27 and 57 years of age leads them to conclude that 'declines in functioning, particularly in memory, in older mildly and moderately mentally retarded adults with DS are not a necessary occurrence within the age range sampled' (Devenny *et al.* 1992).

Other studies, however, report a loss of learning and memory capacities that seems to affect most areas of cognitive function in ageing individuals with DS (Caltagirone *et al.* 1990), although not in a uniform way. Language seemed particularly impaired in this latter study of subjects with a mean age of about 35 years, and the profile that was observed was not the same as that seen in AD. Hemdal *et al.* (1993), on the other hand, report that a group of subjects with mean age of about 24 years had deficits in olfactory identification that seemed quite like that observed in AD. Similarly, Woodruff-Pak *et al.* (1995) showed that DS subjects older than 35 years of age were likely to have deficits in eyeblink conditioning similar to that observed in patients with AD. This latter result is perhaps indicative of defective cerebellar functioning.

Ellis *et al.* (1989) tested a group of subjects with a mean age of 26.8 years on a task that assessed memory for pictures, and for their location in a book. These subjects were very poor on recall of the pictures and also significantly worse on remembering their location. Interestingly, there was a bimodal distribution of the subjects with DS – some did quite well on the location task, while others did very poorly.

Overall, there is evidence from the study of older individuals with DS consistent with the view that their learning and memory deficits are not across-the-board. However, there are not enough data to make precise statements about what is more impaired and what is less impaired. There is also evidence that in old age, as in infancy and childhood, there is a very wide range of possible outcomes. The fact that with ageing there is an increasing possibility that individuals with DS will develop cognitive signs similar to, if not identical with, Alzheimer's disease, certainly suggests that there must be some underlying similarities in their neuropathological profiles. The fact that many older individuals with DS do not develop a full-blown Alzheimer's profile is cause for hope and also cause to be cautious before accepting too quickly the view that these syndromes are largely identical in old age.

## 2.5 Conclusions

Learning and memory are disrupted in Down's syndrome, but we still do not have a precise way of defining exactly what the deficit is. Most indications suggest that the impairment is not spread across all learning and memory systems equally, but instead selectively impacts on some systems. In this regard, the learning and memory systems involving the hippocampus and entorhinal cortex are prime suspects.

Our review of neuropathology suggests that major differences between normally-developing children and those with DS emerge only some months after birth. The corollary to this is the relatively normal, though restricted, learning observed in early infancy. Important deficits emerge within the first year, and they take on a very specific character. There are deficits in learning specific kinds of information, such as about places, or particular features of language, and there are deficits of a more abstract nature, such as the apparent instability of material that has apparently been learned, only to be 'forgotten' shortly thereafter.

Throughout childhood and adolescence serious learning impairments exist, restricting the level of achievement of the vast majority of individuals with DS to a very modest level. At this stage, one sees considerable instability, as well as long periods of time during which little or no progress is made, only to be followed by new acquisitions. At the same time, there are exceptions to this pattern, individuals who achieve considerable heights, and whose progress holds out hope for the future. Much remains to be done before we have a clear understanding of learning and memory capacities in young individuals with DS. Careful studies of various kinds of learning are needed, preferably guided by knowledge of the different learning and memory systems in the brain.

With advancing years, there is a virtual certainty that individuals with DS will develop neuropathology that looks like that seen in AD. However, it is now well documented that only a portion of these subjects will actually develop the dementia characteristic of Alzheimer's. Though there is as yet no accepted explanation for this uncoupling of the neuropathology and dementia, it is a fact of considerable practical and theoretical importance. The most recent neuropsychological work only strengthens the view that there is some critical difference between the two. Determining why a large proportion of individuals with DS apparently avoid the sequella of AD is an important task for research in the coming years.

To sum up, we are slowly unravelling the enigma that is the mental retardation associated with DS. Knowledge of which learning systems are particular affected, and which preferentially spared, will help in the design of more effective early intervention programmes. If current indications that the hippocampal system is particularly subject to disruption hold up, this might suggest approaching children with DS in a way not unlike that used with amnesic patients (Glisky and Schacter 1989), that is, by concentrating on learning and memory systems that are more or less intact. Two advantages of this approach are, firstly, that the children would experience success rather than frustration much of the time, and secondly, that it might be possible to build on the knowledge gained through these systems to acquire skills usually dependent on the other systems. On the other hand, early stimulation of the at-risk hippocampal system (and possibly cerebellar system as well) could both improve its status in infancy and childhood as well as diminish the likelihood of AD-like neuropathology with ageing. There are thus good reasons to focus on both sides of the equation, and to approach intervention with due regard to the complex nature of the learning and memory deficit.

## Acknowledgements

This chapter was written while the author was on a sabbatical from, and supported by, the University of Arizona. Support for this work was also provided by the Cognitive Neuroscience Program grants from the McDonnell Foundation and the Flinn Foundation.

## Notes

1. It seems entirely probable that for most characteristics, including mental functions, there is a 'normal' distribution of values – a typical bell curve – in both normally developing infants and infants with DS.
2. Although this interpretation of inefficiency makes intuitive sense, it does make one pause for a moment in thinking about results from *all* PET studies, in which increases in activity are usually interpreted as signs of normal, not inefficient, function.
3. In an intriguing study of perceptual capacity, Bihrle *et al.* (1989) have shown that adolescents with DS are considerably more impaired in analysis of local features as compared with global features. This result strongly points to the inferotemporal cortex, and perhaps more precisely to the dorsal region (see Horel 1994, for an analysis of the role of this area in local *v.* global perception).
4. Results from the study of an animal model of DS, the trisomy-16 mouse, are consistent with this emphasis upon the hippocampus. Cultured hippocampal neurons from this preparation were shown to have abnormal electrical properties, which could influence hippocampal development (Galdzicki *et al.* 1993).

## References


Ball MJ and Nuttall K (1981) Topography of neurofibrillary tangles and granovacuoles in the hippocampi of patients with Down's syndrome: Quantitative comparison with normal ageing and Alzheimer's disease. Neuropathology and Applied Neurobiology 7: 13–20.

Ball MJ, Schapiro MB and Rapoport SI (1986) Neuropathological relationships between Down syndrome and senile dementia Alzheimer type. In CJ Epstein (Ed) The neurobiology of Down syndrome, pp.45–58. New York: Raven Press.

Bar-Peled O, Israeli M, Ben-Hur H, Hoskins I, Groner Y and Biegon A (1991) Developmental patterns of muscarinic receptors in normal and Down's syndrome fetal brain – an autoradiographic study. Neuroscience Letters 133: 154–8.

Becker LE, Armstrong DL and Chan F (1986) Dendritic atrophy in children with Down's syndrome. Annals of Neurology 20: 520–6.

Benda CE (1971) Mongolism. In J Minckler (Ed) Pathology of the nervous system 2: 1867. New York: McGraw-Hill.

Bihrle AM, Bellugi U, Delis D and Marks S (1989) Seeing the forest for the trees: Dissociation in visuospatial processing. Brain and Cognition 11: 37–49.

Blackwood W and Corsellis JAN (1976) Greenfield's neuropathology, pp.420–1. Chicago: Yearbook Medical.

Brooksbank BWL, Walker D, Balazs R and Jorgensen OS (1989) Neuronal maturation in the foetal brain in Down syndrome. Early Human Development 18: 237–46.

Caltagirone C, Nocentini U and Vicari S (1990) Cognitive functions in adult Down's syndrome. International Journal of Neuroscience 54: 221–30.

Cohen NJ and Eichenbaum H (1993) Memory, amnesia, and the hippocampal system. Cambridge MA: MIT Press.

Cohen NJ and Squire LR (1980) Preserved learning and retention of a patter-analyzing skill in amnesia: Dissociation of knowing how and knowing that. Science 210: 207–10.

Cole G, Neal JW, Singhrao SK, Jasani B and Newman GR (1993) The distribution of amyloid plaques in the cerebellum and brain stem in Down's syndrome and

Alzheimer's disease: a light microscopical analysis. Acta Neuropathologica 85: 542–52.

Cork LC (1990) Neuropathology of Down syndrome and Alzheimer disease. American Journal of Medical Genetics Supplement 7: 282–6.

Courage ML, Adams RJ, Reyno S and Kwa P-G (1994) Visual acuity in infants and children with Down syndrome. Developmental Medicine and Child Neurology 36: 586–93.

Crome L, Cowie V and Slater E (1966) A statistical note on cerebellar and brain-stem weight in Mongolism. Journal of Mental Deficiency 10: 69–72.

Deb S, de Silva PN, Gemmell, HG, Besson JAO, Smith FW and Ebmeier KP (1992) Alzheimer's disease in adults with Down's syndrome: the relationship between regional cerebral blood flow equivalents and dementia. Acta Psychiatrica Scandinavica 86: 340–5.

Devenny DA, Hill AL, Patxot O, Silverman WP and Wisniewski KE (1992) Ageing in higher functioning adults with Down's syndrome: an interim report in a longitudinal study. Journal of Intellectual Disability Research 36: 241–50.

Devinsky O, Sato S, Conwit RA and Schapiro MB (1990) Relation of EEG alpha background to cognitive function, brain atrophy, and cerebral metabolism in Down's syndrome. Archives of Neurology 47: 58–62.

Ellis NR, Woodley-Zanthos P and Dulaney CL (1989) Memory for spatial location in children, adults, and mentally retarded persons. American Journal on Mental Retardation 93: 521–7.

Ferrer I and Gullotta F (1990) Down's syndrome and Alzheimer's disease: dendritic spine counts in hippocampus. Acta Neuropathologica 79: 680–5.

Florez J, del Arco C, Gonzalez A, Pascual J and Pazos A (1990) Autoradiographic studies of neurotransmitter receptors in the brain of newborn infants with Down syndrome. American Journal of Medical Genetics Supplement 7: 301–5.

Fowler A (1988) Determinants of rate of language growth in children with DS. In L Nadel (Ed) The psychobiology of Down syndrome, pp.215–45. Cambridge MA: MIT Press.

Galdzicki Z, Coan E and Rapoport SI (1993) Cultured hippocampal neurons from trisomy 16 mouse, a model for Down's syndrome, have an abnormal action potential due to a reduced inward sodium current. Brain Research 604: 69–78.

Gibson D and Harris A (1988) Aggregated early intervention effects for Down's syndrome persons: patterning and longevity of benefits. Journal of Mental Deficiency Research 32: 1–17.

Glisky EL and Schacter DL (1989) Extending the limits of complex learning in organic amnesia: Computer training in a vocational domain. Neuropsychologia 27: 107–20.

Haier RJ, Chueh D, Touchette P, Lott I, MacMillan D, Sandman C, LaCasse L, Friedman G and Sosa E (1995) Brain size and cerebral glucose metabolic rate in non-specific mental retardation and Down syndrome. Manuscript submitted for publication.

Hemdal P, Corwin J and Oster H (1993) Olfactory identification deficits in Down's syndrome and idiopathic mental retardation. Neuropsychologia 31: 977–84.

Henderson SE (1985) Motor skill development. In D Lane and B Stratford (Eds) Current approaches to Down's syndrome, pp.187–218. Eastbourne UK: Holt Rinehart and Winston.

Hepper PG, and Shahidullah S (1992) Habituation in Normal and Down's syndrome fetuses. The Quarterly Journal of Experimental Psychology 44B: 305–17.

Hopmann MR and Nothnagle MB (1994 April) A longitudinal study of early vocabulary of infants with Down syndrome and infants who are developing normally. Poster presented at the International Down Syndrome Research Conference. Charleston S.

Horel J (1994) Local and global perception examined by reversible suppression of temporal cortex with cold. Behavioural Brain Research 65: 157–64.

Horwitz B, Schapiro MB, Grady CL and Rapoport SI (1990) Cerebral metabolic pattern in young adult Down's syndrome subject: altered intercorrelations between regional rates of glucose utilization. Journal of Mental Deficiency Research 34: 237–52.

Hyman BT (1992) Down syndrome and Alzheimer disease. In L Nadel and CJ Epstein (Eds) Down syndrome and Alzheimer disease, pp.123–42. New York: Wiley-Liss.

Jernigan TL and Bellugi U (1990) Anomolous brain morphology on magnetic resonance images in Williams syndrome and Down syndrome. Archive of Neurology 47: 529–33.

Jiang ZD, Wu YY and Liu XY (1990) Early development in brainstem auditory evoked potentials in Down's syndrome. Early Human Development 23: 41–51.

Kesslak JP, Nagata SF, Lott I and Nalcioglu O (1994) Magnetic resonance imaging analysis of age-related changes in the brains of individuals with Down's syndrome. Neurology 44: 1039-45.

Lynch M, Oller D, Steffens M and Buder E (in press) Phrasing in prelinguistic vocalizations. Development Psychology.

Mangan PA (1992) Spatial memory abilities and abnormal development in the hippocampal formation in Down syndrome. Unpublished doctoral dissertation. University of Arizona, Tucson.

Mangan PA and Nadel L (1990) Development of spatial memory in human infants. Bulletin of the Psychonomic Society 28: 513.

Mann DMA and Esiri MM (1989) The pattern of acquisition of plaques and tangles in the brains of patients under 50 years of age with Down's syndrome. Journal of the Neurological Sciences 89: 169–79.

Mann DMA, Royston MC and Ravindra CR (1990) Some morphometric observations on the brains of patients with Down's syndrome: their relationship to age and dementia. Journal of the Neurological Sciences 99: 153–64.

Marcell MM and Cohen S (1992) Hearing abilities of Down synndrome and other mentally handicapped adolescents. Research in Developmental Disabilities 13: 533–51.

McAlaster R (1992) Postnatal cerebral maturation in Down's syndrome children: A developmental EEG coherence study. International Journal of Neuroscience 65: 221-37.

McClelland JL, McNaughton BL, O'Reilly R and Nadel L (1992 May) Complementary roles of the hippocampus and neocortex in learning and memory. Society for Neuroscience. Anaheim CA.

Mishkin M, Malamut B and Bachevalier J (1984) Memories and habits: Two neural systems. In JL McGaugh G Lynch and NM Weinberger (Eds) The neurobiology of learning and memory, pp.65–77. New York: Guildford Press.

Murphy Jr GM, Ellis WG, Lee Y-L, Stultz KE, Shrivastava R, Tinklenberg JR and Eng LF (1992) Astrocytic gliosis in the amygdala in Down's syndrome and Alzheimer's disease. In ACH Yu, L Hertz, MD Norenberg, E Sykova and SG Waxman (Eds) Progress in Brain Research 94: 475–83. Amsterdam: Elsevier.

Murphy Jr GM and Ellis WG (1991) The amygdala in Down's syndrome and familial Alzheimer's disease: Four clinicopathological case reports. Biological Psychiatry 30: 92–106.

Nadel L (1986) Down syndrome in neurobiological perspective. In CJ Epstein (Ed) The neurobiology of Down syndrome, pp. 239–51. New York: Raven Press.

Nadel L (1992) Multiple memory systems: What and why. Journal of Cognitive Neuroscience 4: 179–88.

Nadel L (1994) Multiple memory systems: What and why. An Update. In D Schacter and E Tulving (Eds) Memory Systems 1994, pp. 39–63. Cambridge MA: MIT Press.

Nadel L and O'Keefe J (1974) The hippocampus in pieces and patches: an essay on modes of explanation in physiological psychology. In R Bellairs and EG Gray (Eds) Essays on the nervous system. A Festschrift for JZ Young, pp.367–90. Oxford: The Clarendon Press.

Nadel L and Willner J (1989) Some implications of postnatal maturation in the hippocampal formation. In V Chan-Palay and C. Köhler (Eds) The hippocampus: new vistas, pp.17–31. New York: Liss.

Nadel L and Zola-Morgan S (1984) Infantile amnesia: a neurobiological perspective. In M Moscovitch (Ed) Infant memory, pp.111–31. New York: Plenum Press.

Nelson L, Lott I, Touchette P, Satz P and D'Elia L (in press) Detection of Alzheimer's disease in persons with Down's syndrome: Possible relevance of depression. American Journal on Mental Retardation.

Ohr PS and Fagen JW (1991) Conditioning and long-term memory in three-month-old infants with Down syndrome. American Journal on Mental Retardation 96: 151–62.

Ohr PS and Fagen JW (1993) Temperament, conditioning, and memory in 3-month-old infants with Down syndrome. Journal of Applied Developmental Psychology 14: 175–90.

Ohr PS and Fagen JW (1994) Contingency learning in 9-month-old infants with Down syndrome. American Journal on Mental Retardation 99: 74–84.

O'Keefe J and Nadel L (1978) The hippocampus as a cognitive map. Oxford: The Clarendon Press.

Pazos A, del Olmo E, Diaz A, del Arco C, Rodriguez-Puertas R, Pascual J, Palacios JM and Florez J (1994 April) Serotonergic (5-$HT_{1A}$ and 5-$HT_{1D}$) and muscarinic cholinergic receptors in DS brains: An autoradiographic analysis. Poster presented at the International Down Syndrome Research Conference, Charleston SC.

Poulson CL (1988) Operant conditioning of vocalization rate of infants with Down syndrome. American Journal on Mental Retardation 93: 57–63.

Raz N, Torres IJ, Briggs SD, Spencer WD, Thornton AE, Loken WJ, Gunning FM, McQuain JD, Driesen NR and Acker JD (in press) Selective neuroanatomical abnormalities in Down syndrome and their cognitive correlates: Evidence from MRI morphometry. Neurology.

Rondal JA (1994) Exceptional language development in mental retardation: The relative autonomy of language as a cognitive system. In H Tager-Flusberg (Ed) Constraints on language acquisition: Studies of atypical children, pp.155–74. Hillsdale NJ: Erlbaum.

Schacter DL and Tulving E (1994) Memory systems 1994. Cambridge MA: MIT Press.

Schapiro MB, Haxby JV and Grady CL (1992) Nature of mental retardation and dementia in Down syndrome: Study with PET, CT, and neuropsychology. Neurobiology of Aging 13: 723–34.

Schmidt-Sidor B, Wisniewski K, Shepard TH and Sersen EA (1990) Brain growth in Down syndrome subjects 15 to 22 weeks of gestational age and birth to 60 months. Clinical Neuropathology 9: 181–90.

Spargo E, Luthert PJ, Janota I and Lantos PL (1992) β4A deposition in the temporal cortex of adults with Down's syndrome. Journal of the Neurological Sciences 111: 26–32.

Squire LR (1992) Memory and the hippocampus: A synthesis of findings with rats, monkeys, and humans. Psychological Review 99: 195–231.

Squire LR, Cohen NJ and Nadel L (1984) The medial temporal region and memory consolidation: A new hypothesis. In H Weingartner and E Parker (Eds) Memory consolidation, pp.185–210, Hillsdale NJ: Erlbaum.

Sutherland RJ and Rudy JW (1989) Configural association theory: The role of the hippocampal formation in learning, memory, and amnesia. Psychobiology 17: 129–44.

Sylvester PE (1983) The hippocampus in Down's syndrome. Journal of Mental Deficiency Research 27: 227–36.

Uecker A, Obrzut JE and Nadel L (1994) Mental rotation performance by learning disabled and Down's syndrome children: A study of imaginal development. Developmental Neuropsychology 10: 395–411.

Weis S (1991) Morphometry and magnetic resonance imaging of the human brain in normal controls and Down's syndrome. The Anatomical Record 231: 593–8.

Wishart J (1993) The development of learning difficulties in children with Down syndrome. Journal of Intellectual Disability Research 37: 389–403.

Wisniewski KE, Laure-Kamionowska M, Connell F and Wen GY (1986) Neuronal density and synaptogenesis in the postnatal stage of brain maturation in Down syndrome. In CJ Epstein (Ed) The neurobiology of Down syndrome, pp.29–44. New York: Raven Press.

Wisniewski K and Schmidt-Sidor B (1989) Postnatal delay of myelin formation in brains from Down syndrome infants and children. Clinical Neuropathology 8: 55–62.

Woodruff-Pak DS, Papka M and Simon EW (1995) Down's syndrome adults aged 35 and older show eyeblink classical conditioning profiles comparable to Alzheimer's disease patients. Manuscript submitted for publication.

# 3
# Alzheimer's Disease, Neuropathology and Dementia in Down's Syndrome

**HENRYK M WISNIEWSKI AND WAYNE SILVERMAN**

## 3.1 Introduction

Alzheimer's disease (AD) is the most common cause of old-age associated dementia, with current projections indicating, for example, that over 2 million Americans will have this disease by the year 2000 (Rocca *et al.* 1986). Adults with Down's syndrome (DS) are particularly vulnerable to this devastating disease (see Zigman *et al.* 1993, for a recent review).

*Clinically*, AD follows a predictable progression, although significant individual heterogeneity has been noted (Reisberg 1983). Onset of symptoms is insidious, with the earliest stages characterized by mild disturbances of recent memory. *Agnosia* (deficits in processing of sensory information with no peripheral impairment), *aphasia* (expressive language difficulty) and *apraxia* (motor performance deficits with normally functioning sensory and musculoskeletal systems) are characteristic of the progressive AD dementia. Adaptive skills will deteriorate, and eventually the most basic skills are lost (e.g., dependence in toileting and eating). Eventually, if an affected individual does not succumb to a competing cause of death, AD will result in a totally vegetative state characterized by the complete loss of motor, language and self-care skills.

The rate of progression of the disease varies across individuals. Nevertheless, while promising palliatives are currently being tested, no treatment of the underlying pathology is available at present and the progression of dementia is inevitable.

*Neuropathologically*, AD is characterized by a broad spectrum of brain changes. These include:

1. Gross atrophy;
2. Synapse and neuronal loss;
3. Formation of β-amyloid plaques of various composition (primitive,

classical, diffuse);
4. Formation of neurofibrillary tangles within neurons;
5. Amyloid angiopathy;
6. Granulovacuolar degeneration;
7. Presence of Hirano bodies.

Plaques and tangles are considered the neuropathological hallmarks of AD, and are present in significantly higher densities in the neocortex in AD compared with 'normal' ageing. These lesions can be observed in smaller numbers in 'normal' brains, and therefore diagnosis is dependent upon quantitative, rather than qualitative criteria.

Diagnosis of AD is a difficult and involved task that relies on the presence of both clinical symptoms and specific neuropathological changes (Reisberg 1983; Wisniewski *et al.* 1989). Dementia is a symptomatic diagnosis that requires systematic documentation of progressive deterioration over an extended period of time. Because the cause of AD is unknown and many other conditions can cause a dementing syndrome, AD currently is diagnosed clinically by exclusion of alternative causes in conjunction with documentation of a pattern of dementia consistent with this disease. However, even with the best clinical evaluation, definitive diagnosis requires neuropathological confirmation, and the clearest clinical profile provides the basis only for a 'probable' identification of AD.

The diagnostic complexities associated with a definitive diagnosis of AD in the general population are amplified for adults with mental retardation, and especially for adults with DS. With respect to dementia, the diagnostic criteria and methodology developed for use with the non-retarded population assumes a premorbid level of functioning that adults with mental retardation have never achieved. In addition, the limited expressive communication skills of many adults with mental retardation, and especially those with DS, can make assessment of early changes associated with AD extremely difficult to identify. Finally, given the lifelong differences in the experiences of most adults with mental retardation compared with their non-retarded peers, it is likely that AD changes will present atypically (Barcikowska *et al.* 1989). Therefore, diagnosis of dementia requires careful objective documentation of decreasing performance levels over an extended period of time, measured against premorbid baselines established for each individual. Of course, given the wide variability in baseline performance across individuals, this means that different assessment batteries are likely to be needed for people with mild, moderate, severe and profound mental retardation, although the newest classification system recommends that these terms no longer be used (AAMR 1992).

Once dementia has been identified, differential diagnosis of AD requires alternative causes to be ruled out. This can be a difficult process, especially for adults with DS, who are likely to present with a combination of symptoms (Seltzer and Luchterhand 1994), including atypical thyroid function and depression (Burt *et al.* 1992). As in the case of AD, clinical presentation of these co-morbid conditions also can be atypical, and even when diagnosed correctly, responses to interventions can vary substantially from case to case. For example, it seems clear that non-responsiveness to antidepressants cannot be a definitive criterion for ruling out suspected depression in this population, and diagnosis of AD should be delayed until all intervention options have been exhausted. This is necessarily a long and involved process.

Finally, for adults with DS the interpretation of neuropathological findings, currently the definitive diagnostic criteria, is complicated by the fact that virtually all adults with DS over 40 years of age that have been evaluated have exceeded neuropathological criteria for AD, whether or not a history of dementia can be documented (Malamud 1972; Khachaturian 1985). Thus, the best and most objective indicators of AD in populations without DS (presence of many plaques and tangles) do not discriminate reliably between demented and non-demented adults with DS.

Given this background, we will now discuss our current understanding of AD within the population of adults with DS and describe some recent findings that contribute to clarification of some key issues of debate.

## 3.2 Recent Findings

As mentioned above, neuropathology consistent with a diagnosis of AD has been observed in virtually all cases of adults with DS over the age of 40 that have received postmortem evaluation (see Zigman *et al.* 1993, for a recent review). Thus, there is overwhelming neuropathological evidence that this population is susceptible to AD with precocious onset (Mann 1988). Other recent evidence from molecular studies of chromosome 21 have indicated that genes present in triplicate in people with DS play important roles in AD pathogenesis (Goldgaber *et al.* 1987; Robakis *et al.* 1987; Tanzi *et al.* 1987).

In contrast to the consistent picture that emerges from studies of AD neuropathology among adults with DS, clinical studies show wide variation in the prevalence of dementia (Zigman *et al.* 1993). Only a single study has found dementia in 100% of cases (Lott and Lai 1982), and it is impossible to generalize from this sample, because it consisted exclusively of cases referred for suspected mental deterioration. Typically, studies of dementia find a minority of positive cases, even at ages over 50. In fact, Devenny et al. (1992) are currently following 90 adults with DS and mild/moderate mental retardation prospectively and are finding possible dementia of the Alzheimer type in very few individuals ($n = 7$).

The largest longitudinal study conducted to date, Zigman *et al.* (in press) examined change over time in adults with mental retardation of all levels, including individuals residing in both community and institutional settings. Detailed analyses indicated that relative risk for decline in adaptive skills is comparable among adults with and without DS until they reach 50 years of age. After 50, relative risk increases significantly for adults with DS compared with their peers without DS (matched on age and level of mental retardation), but even after 60, risk did not approach 100%.

Of course, this suggests a major discrepancy between the presumed presence of AD-type neuropathological changes, which appear to begin at around 30-35 years of age in adults with DS, and clinical dementia, which seems undetectable in many adults even 30 years later.

The first possible explanation for this discrepancy is associated with the imprecision of clinical diagnosis. It would not be surprising for early stages of AD dementia to go unrecognized in this population because adults with DS are likely:

(a) to present with atypical symptoms;
(b) to have lifelong impairments that limit the utility of standard assessment methods and criteria;
(c) to have co-morbid conditions that can account for changes in status;
(d) to exhibit many characteristics of precocious but otherwise 'normal' ageing.

Nevertheless, despite difficulties with early identification of dementia, there is a consensus that end-stage disease is clearly recognizable except in cases with profound MR and multiple handicaps. Therefore, it seems unlikely that diagnostic insensitivity can account totally for the disparity between clinical and neuropathological profiles. Given that it is unusual to observe a clinical course of AD in the non-retarded population that exceeds 20 years (Reisberg 1983), it seems extremely unlikely that in the DS population, where individuals are prone to precocious ageing generally and onset of AD specifically, a slower rate of progression would be expected, but this assumption must be made to explain current data based solely upon reference to false negative clinical evaluation.

As a second possible explanation for the disparity described above, investigators have suggested that something within the DS brain provides a compensatory mechanism that counteracts the effects of the advancing neuropathology for a prolonged period of time until some threshold associated with clinical manifestation is reached (Wisniewski and Rabe 1986). However, the reduced neural densities characteristic of the DS brain suggest that, if anything, fewer compensatory mechanisms should be available to these individuals compared with their non-retarded peers.

We suggest that a third explanation for the apparent disparity between clinical and neuropathological profiles of AD in adults with DS is available. This explanation is supported by recent detailed studies of AD neuropathology, primarily based upon quantitative studies of immunocytochemically treated material. As discussed earlier, abundant formation of β-amyloid plaques occurs in the brains of adults with DS as early as in their teens (Mann 1988). However, not all plaques are equivalent. For present purposes, two classes of plaques will be distinguished: (a) those associated with fibrillization and (b) those that do not contain fibrils. Both classes of plaques contain β-amyloid protein, and both are stained by antibodies to β-amyloid as well as some silver techniques. However, non-fibrillar plaques are formed at earlier ages than are fibrillar, or neuritic plaques, and only this latter class of plaques appears to be associated with clinical dementia. This has been noted previously for non-retarded adults with AD (Braak and Braak 1992), and now in our studies of DS (Wisniewski *et al.* 1995). In fact, we have shown that non-fibrillized plaques are observed in people with DS as young as 16, while densities of fibrillized plaques are not characteristic of cases until their 40s and up, with a significant increase in densities of these plaques observed after individuals reach 50 years of age.

From additional studies, our results indicate that the cellular origin of these two subclasses of β-amyloid plaques may be different (Wisniewski and Wegiel 1995). Specifically, neurons appear to produce diffuse, non-fibrillar plaques while microglia and perivascular cells appear to produce fibrillar plaques. We suggest that it is the fibrillar plaques that are associated with the disruption of normal neural functioning. Therefore, formation of these 'malignant' fibrillar plaques, plus the concomitant development of neurofibrillary tangles, would be the critical events that lead to the cascade of brain changes underlying Alzheimer's disease and the associated dementia.

If this is proven to be correct, the disparity between the clinical and neuropathological profiles of AD among adults with DS can be explained. Routine neuropathological evaluations do not differentiate well between fibrillized and non-fibrillized plaques, and while a considerable β-amyloid burden can be present in adults with DS in their 30s, this amyloid is in the non-fibrillar, benign form. It is not until some 20 years later that we see significant accumulations of fibrillized plaques.

Of course, if this were the sole mechanism determining AD dementia, then virtually all individuals with DS would be exhibiting dementia by their late 50s or early 60s. This is clearly not the case (see Devenny *et al.* 1992; Zigman *et al.* in press; and Zigman *et al.* 1993, for recent reviews). Multiple factors must determine vulnerability, as suggested recently by Khachaturian (in press) and Wisniewski *et al.* (1995). We can conceptualize onset of disease determined by an 'AND' gate, as indicated in Figure 3.1. Genetic factors, such as increased amyloid load in DS associated with triplication of the amyloid precursor protein gene on chromosome 21, an APP point mutation, or a predisposing form of APOE, can increase the probability of age-specific disease onset, as can various environmental exposures. In addition, chronological age and individual rates of ageing will affect age at onset, and these three broad categories of factors act in conjunction to determine age of onset, and perhaps rate of progression.

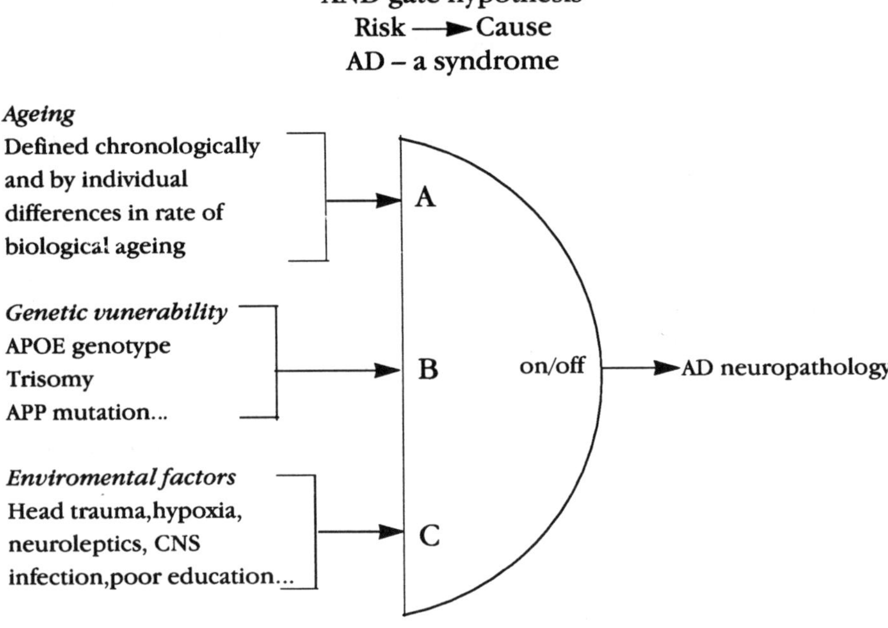


*Figure 3.1* Schematic illustration of multiple determinants of age-specific risk for Alzheimer's disease.

## 3.3 Conclusions

For adults with DS, this is a much more positive picture than has been broadly accepted in the recent past. Neuropathologists have been thinking about AD as an inevitable consequence of trisomy 21, but it now appears that onset is much later than has been estimated by classical studies, and that the presumed disparity between clinical and neuropathological manifestations of this terrible disease can be explained, not by assuming that symptoms go unrecognized, but by understanding that an extended period of asymptomatic benign brain amyloidosis occurs. Someday, this benign period of 20 plus years may provide an opportunity for effective intervention that could prevent the onset of a dementing syndrome.

Our results suggest that the β-amyloid precursor protein gene dose effect causes the occurrence of early diffuse plaques. However, other as yet unspecified ageing genes that appear to be on chromosome 21 could be as important in making adults with DS vulnerable to many age-associated changes, including Alzheimer's disease, some 20 to 30 years prematurely. Multiple other factors that control individual rates of ageing, APP processing, and neurofibrillary tangle formation will determine which adults with DS will exhibit signs and symptoms of dementia at any given age. This hypothesis is supported by our recent studies of neurofibrillary changes in brains of adults with DS showing great variation in individual susceptibility to neurofibrillary pathology among these persons (Wegiel *et al.* 1996). This reasoning leads us to predict that the age-specific risk for Alzheimer's disease among adults with Down's syndrome should look remarkably similar to that of the general population, but with an earlier age of onset.

## Acknowledgements

Supported by funds provided by New York State through its Office of Mental Retardation and Developmental Disabilities, as well as Grant Nos. PO1 AG11531 and PO1 AG04220 from the National Institute on Ageing.

## References

American Association on Mental Retardation (1992) Mental retardation: definition, classification and systems of supports. Washington DC: American Association on Mental Retardation.

Barcikowska M, Silverman W, Zigman W, Kozlowski P, Kujawa M, Rudelli R and Wisniewski H (1989) Alzheimer-type neuropathology and clinical symptoms of dementia in mentally retarded people without Down syndrome. American Journal on Mental Retardation 93: 551–7.

Braak H and Braak E (1992) The human entorhinal cortex: normal morphology and lamina-specific pathology in various diseases. Neuroscience Research 15: 6–31.

Burt D, Loveland K and Lewis K (1992) Depression and the onset of dementia in adults with mental retardation. American Journal on Mental Retardation 96: 506–71.

Devenny D, Hill AL, Patxot O, Silverman W and Wisniewski K (1992) Ageing in higher functioning adults with Down syndrome: an interim report of a longitudinal study. Journal of Mental Deficiency Research 36: 241–50.

Goldgaber D, Lerman M, McBride O, Saffiotti V and Gajdusek D (1987) Characterization and chromosomal localization of a cDNA encoding brain amyloid of Alzheimer's disease. Science 235: 877–80.

Khachaturian Z (1985) Diagnosis of Alzheimer's disease. Archives of Neurology 42: 1097–105.

Khachaturian Z (in press) Calcium hypothesis of Alzheimer's disease and brain aging. Annals New York Academy of Sciences.

Lott I and Lai F (1982) Dementia in Down syndrome: observations from a neurology clinic. Applied Research in Mental Retardation 3: 233–9.

Malamud N (1972) Neuropathology of organic brain syndromes associated with aging. In CM Gaitz (Ed) Aging and the brain, pp.63–87. New York: Plenum.

Mann D (1988) The pathological association between Down's syndrome and Alzheimer's disease. Mechanisms in Aging and Development 43: 99–136.

Reisberg B (1983) Clinical presentation, diagnosis and symptomatology of age-associated cognitive decline and Alzheimer's disease. In B Reisberg (Ed) Alzheimer's disease: the standard reference, pp.173–87. New York: Free Press.

Robakis N, Wisniewski H, Jenkins EC, Devine-Gage E, Houck G, Yao X, Ramakrishna N, Wolfe G, Silverman W and Brown WT (1987) Chromosome 21q21 sublocalization of gene encoding beta-amyloid peptide in cerebral vessels and neuritic (senile) plaques of people with Alzheimer's disease and Down syndrome. Lancet 1: 384–5.

Rocca W, Amaducci L and Schoenberg B (1986) Epidemiology of clinically diagnosed Alzheimer's disease. Annals of Neurology 19: 415–24.

Seltzer G and Luchterhand C (1994) Health and well-being of older persons with developmental disabilities: a clinical review. In M Seltzer, M Wyngaarden Kraus and M Janicki (Eds) Life course perspectives on adulthood and old age, pp.109–42. Washington DC: American Association on Mental Retardation.

Tanzi R, Gusella J, Watkins P, Bruns G, St. George-Hyslop P, Van Keuren M, Patterson S, Jurnit D, Neve R (1987) Amyloid β protein gene: cDNA mRNA distribution, and genetic linkage near the Alzheimer locus. Science 285: 880–4.

Wegiel J, Wisniewski HM, Dziewiatkowski J, Popovitch ER and Tarnawski M (in press) Differential susceptibililty to neurofibrillary pathology among patients with Down syndrome.

Wisniewski H and Rabe A (1986) Discrepancy between Alzheimer-type neuropathology and dementia in persons with Down syndrome. Annals of the New York Academy of Sciences 477: 247–59.

Wisniewski HM, Rabe A, Zigman W and Silverman W (1989) Editorial. Neuropathological diagnosis of Alzheimer disease. Journal of Neuropathological Experimental Neurology 48: 606–9.

Wisniewski H and Wegiel J (1995) Alzheimer disease and the pathogenesis of beta and paired helical filament (tau) protein fibrillization. In K Iqbal, J Mortimer, B Winblad and H Wisniewski (Eds) Research advances in Alzheimer's disease and related disorders, pp. 569–575. New York: Wiley.

Wisniewski H, Wegiel J and Popovitch E (1995) Age-associated development of diffuse and thioflavin-S-positive plaques in Down syndrome. Developmental Brain Dysfunction 7: 330–9.

Zigman W, Schupf N, Sersen E and Silverman W (1996) Prevalence of dementia in adults with and without Down syndrome. American Journal on Mental Retardation 100, 403–12.

Zigman W, Schupf N, Zigman A and Silverman W (1993) Aging and Alzheimer disease in people with mental retardation. In N Bray (Ed) International review of research in mental retardation 19: 41–70. New York: Academic Press.

# Part Two: Perception and Cognition

# 4

# Visual and Auditory Perception in Children with Down's Syndrome

SIEGFRIED M. PUESCHEL AND MARIA SUSTROVA

## 4.1 Introduction

All information about the world comes to us by the way of our senses. In order to gather information from the environment, every human being has to use his/her vision, hearing, smell, taste and tactile senses. Thus, by means of our sensory experiences, we learn from our surroundings and – using Piagetian terminology – processes of assimilation and accommodation take place. According to Piaget, these two processes are the primary means by which children learn to know about objects and situations either by assimilating the object to an already existing scheme, or by accommodating that scheme to the object at hand.

Many psychologists have focused on sensory processing and perception in children. In particular, Piaget has made a significant contribution in the realm of perception psychology. There are also numerous other investigators who have pursued important work in the area of perception and how sensory experiences affect human functioning.

An in-depth review of the literature reveals that there are voluminous data on the subject of visual and auditory processing. Within the framework of this paper, we will only be able to discuss a mere fraction of the available information as it relates to persons with Down's syndrome.

## 4.2 Biologic Concerns of Visual and Auditory Functioning

Before we engage in a discussion of visual and auditory perception in children with Down's syndrome (DS), we would like to briefly focus on the importance of the organic aspects of the sensory systems. If we do not have adequate vision and auditory functioning, because of underlying structural defects or other significant pathology, then optimal visual and auditory perception cannot take place.

### 4.2.1 Ophthalmologic disorders

Concerning ophthalmologic aspects in children with DS, it is well known that a number of ocular disorders are observed at a higher frequency in children with DS. For example, strabismus has been noted to occur in 20–30% of children with DS. Esotropia is observed more frequently in children with DS, whereas exotropia is found less often. The most important causes of strabismus are lens opacities and uncorrected refractive errors.

Another frequently observed ocular finding is nystagmus which is present in 10–20% of children with DS. It can be the result of a central nervous system lesion or it may be due to a refractive error.

Abnormalities of the cornea include corneal opacities and keratoconus. The latter condition occurs in 2–7% of persons with DS, primarily after puberty. Keratoconus is characterized by an increased curvature of the inferior-temporal central portion of the cornea. Keratoconus may be due to a combination of internal and external factors such as an underlying disorder of connective tissue with additional irritation through rubbing of the eye.

Cataracts are also noted more often in persons with DS than in the general population. Congenital cataracts occur in approximately 3% of newborns. These are usually dense opacities of the lens requiring immediate surgery. In addition, three types of acquired cataracts have been observed in persons with DS: arcuate, sutural and flake opacities. It has been estimated that up to 40–50% of individuals with DS develop cataracts with advancing age. Many of the cataractous changes, however, do not warrant surgical intervention.

Errors of refraction including myopia and hyperopia have been reported at a higher prevalence in persons with DS. About 30–50% of persons with DS are myopic, whereas 20–30% have hyperopia. Most of the refractive errors can be corrected. Amblyopia occurs in about 12% of children with DS.

It is paramount that children with DS undergo ophthalmologic examinations from early childhood on, and that the above described and other ocular abnormalities are treated appropriately so that optimal visual function can be assured (Catalano 1992).

Table 4.1 lists major otolaryngologic concerns in Down's syndrome.

Table 4.1 Otolaryngologic concerns

| |
|---|
| External structural ear anomalies |
| Stenotic ear canal/blocked with cerumen |
| Abnormalities of the tympanic membrane |
| Otitis media |
| Middle ear fluid accumulation |
| Ossicular abnormalities |
| Eustachian tube dysfunction |
| Inner ear abnormalities |

### 4.2.2 Otolaryngologic concerns

Numerous reports in the literature attest to the high frequency of structural abnormalities, infectious processes, and other functional abnormalities within the otologic system often resulting in significant hearing impairment. For example, the ear canals of children with DS are usually small and stenotic; they also may be obstructed with cerumen. The tympanic membranes may be retracted, bulging or sclerotic. The middle ear may reveal an acute or chronic infection, fluid accumulation, and/or ossicular abnormalities. Eustachian tube dysfunction has also been described in children with DS. There may be other anatomic and functional concerns within the otologic system, all of which may result in hearing deficits. It has been reported that up to 80% of children with DS have some form of hearing impairment. Most often, the hearing deficit is due to a conductive hearing loss. There is also an increased prevalence of sensorineural hearing loss in both children and adults with DS.

Because of the high frequency of structural and functional abnormalities of the otologic system, it is important that children with DS be examined regularly, that infections be treated effectively, and structural abnormalities, if possible, be corrected. This will then allow normal auditory perception to take place (Dahle and Baldwin 1992).

## 4.3 Visual Perception in Children with Down's Syndrome

Since the early description of DS in the latter half of the past century, numerous studies have focused on mental abilities in children with this chromosome disorder. In particular, early psychomotor development, genetic influences, biological aspects of central nervous system development, the contribution of environmental factors, and changes in cognitive functioning over time have been discussed in the pertinent literature. However, only a limited number of investigations have been carried out with respect to specific sensory functions in children with DS.

In 1965, Nakamura observed strong visual motor sequencing in subjects with DS. During the same year, Bilovsky and Share (1965) reported that children with DS displayed a relatively strong performance on visual decoding and motor decoding. Similarly, Sackett (1967) reported that individuals with DS exhibited a preference for high visual complexity levels. Gramza and Witt (1969) compared normal preschoolers with children with DS on response to coloured block presentations. Responses for the subjects with DS ranged from non-structured patterning to simple linear and vertical stacking, during which children with DS performed less well than children who did not have this chromosome disorder. In another study (Stratford 1980), 17 individuals with DS were matched on mental age (MA) with 17 children who did not have DS. The subjects were tested on two matching tasks, one involving increasing density of pattern and the other both increasing size and increasing density of pattern. The performance of children with DS was significantly weaker than that of children in the control group who were able to accommodate the imposition of pattern on size.

Miranda and Fantz (1973) studied the differential visual responses of 20 children with DS and those of 20 control infants. Although the subjects with DS looked for a longer time period at the stimuli than the 'normal' children did, they showed a response differential in only three stimulus pairs compared with 11 for the 'normal' infants. Six of the stimulus pairs elicited significant differences between the two groups which were related to the type of stimulus variation. The results of this study point to an early relationship between visual-attentional responses and intellectual potential.

More recently, an Italian group of investigators (Salviolo-Negrin *et al.* 1990) studied visual perceptual abilities and behavioural and social adaptations in 44 subjects with DS. The results indicated a general decline in performance in individuals 25 years and older except in the visual-motor subtest, where a decline was less evident.

Table 4.2 summarizes major findings in the studies reviewed above.

Table 4.2 Selected studies on visual perception in individuals with Down's syndrome

| | |
|---|---|
| Nakamura 1965 | Strength in visual–motor sequencing |
| Bilovsky and Share 1965 | Good visual and motor decoding |
| Sackett 1967 | Preference for high visual complexity |
| Gramza and Witt 1969 | Poor performance stacking coloured blocks |
| Miranda and Fantz 1973 | Visual preference of infants with Down's syndrome |
| Stratford 1980 | Matching for size and density is reduced |
| Salviolo-Negrin *et al.* 1990 | Decline in performance of older persons except in visual motor tasks |

## 4.4 Auditory Perception in Children with Down's Syndrome

Several studies report on auditory preferences, auditory memory, auditory motor channelling, and other auditory processes in persons with DS. Zekulin *et al.* (1974) tested an auditory-motor channelling deficit hypothesis in individuals with DS focusing on modality, distraction and patterning variables. Although the findings of their study did not support the auditory-motor channelling deficit hypothesis, there was evidence that auditory-motor channelling difficulties occur more often in children with DS than in subjects with mental retardation due to other causes.

An interesting study was carried out by Glenn *et al.* (1981) in which 11 infants with DS demonstrated that they could operate an automated device which enabled them to listen to one of a pair of auditory signals. Infants with DS as well as those who did not have this chromosome disorder showed a significant preference for nursery rhymes sung by a female voice rather than played on musical instruments. The infants with DS had much longer response durations for the more complex auditory stimuli than those in the control group.

A different approach was taken by Bowler *et al.* (1985). The authors attempted to resolve the conflicting findings of earlier investigations on the directions of dichotic ear preferences in children with DS. The investigators administered one non-verbal and two verbal dichotic tests to children with DS, and to a group of MA matched nursery school children with average intellectual functioning. Many children with DS had reversed ear advantages for verbal material. This reversal was not found when non-verbal material was used. The authors concluded that reversal of ear advantage for verbal material was not characteristic of children with DS but may be associated with the level of language ability.

Varnhagen *et al.* (1987) studied auditory memory span for letters and component memory processes in young adults with DS. Component processes of the span task included long-term memory access for labels for the stimuli and memory for the order in which the stimuli were presented. The authors indicated that although all subjects had relatively poor auditory memory spans, individuals with DS displayed especially poor long-term memory access for stimulus identification and limited short-term storage for processing of auditory information. Lexical storage and retrieval deficiencies were isolated, accounting for the verbal difficulties experienced by the individuals with DS.

Marcell *et al.* (1988) found that children with DS are susceptible to both auditory distraction and off-task glancing during laboratory tasks. Subjects with DS displayed significantly poorer recall of auditorally presented stimuli than other children who did not have DS. The poor auditory memory of individuals with DS did not improve under testing conditions designed to minimize auditory and visual distractions.

Brainstem auditory-evoked response latencies were investigated by Miezejeski *et al.* (1994). The investigators observed latencies for P3 and P5 which were shorter for individuals with DS than for those in the control groups. The pattern of left versus right ear responses in individuals with DS differed from those in the control groups. Thus, the authors suggested that auditory processing associated with DS is characterized by aberrant lateralization. The degree to which this lateralization differs from that in other individuals who do not have DS may vary along a continuum ranging from clearly opposite asymmetry to a more typical pattern.

Lincoln *et al.* (1985) investigated neurophysiologic correlates of information processing by children with DS. Nine children with DS were compared with two groups of non-retarded children. Event-related brain potential and reaction time results indicated that children with DS process some types of auditory information more slowly than MA matched and chronological age (CA) matched non-retarded children.

Table 4.3 summarizes major findings in the studies reviewed above.

Table 4.3 Selected studies on auditory perception in persons with Down's syndrome

| | | |
|---|---|---|
| Zekulin *et al.* | 1974 | Significant auditory–motor channelling deficits |
| Glenn *et al.* | 1981 | Longer response durations for complex auditory stimuli |
| Bowler *et al.* | 1985 | Reversed ear advantage for verbal stimuli |
| Varnhagen *et al.* | 1987 | Prolonged auditory memory span |
| Marcell *et al.* | 1988 | Decreased recall of auditory stimuli |
| Miezejeski *et al.* | 1994 | Aberrant lateralization of auditory processing |
| Lincoln *et al.* | 1985 | Slow auditory information processing |

## 4.5 Visual and Auditory Processing in Children with Down's Syndrome

There are a few reports in the literature describing both visual and auditory processing deficits in children with DS. For example, Bilovsky and Share (1965) found input–output circuiting to be weakest for the auditory-vocal and strongest for the visual-motor channels. Moreover, Scheffelin (1968) observed auditory-vocal difficulties in children with DS. This author presented paired associates to 24 children with DS who had a mean CA of 11 years and a mean MA of 4 years 6 months. The results revealed that the mean error scores in the visual-motor, visual-vocal, and auditory-motor conditions were similar, but the mean error score in the auditory-vocal condition was approximately twice as large as in the other conditions.

Marcell and Armstrong (1982) studied auditory and visual sequential memory using the Illinois Test of Psycholinguistic Abilities. They found that children with DS had poor auditory sequential memory and marked difficulties recalling auditorally presented verbal material. The authors suggested that the auditory-visual recall difference between subjects with DS and those who do not have this chromosomal abnormality may be due to the differential use of information in echoic memory. Also, Molina and Perez (1993) found that children with DS performed poorly in auditory digit recall tasks. Their study revealed that the auditory-verbal modality is weaker than the visual-motor modality in children with DS.

Auditory and visual digit recall was studied by Marcell (1994) in both children with DS and individuals with mental retardation due to other causes. This investigation suggested that there was modest longitudinal improvement in the overall memory performance for both groups. The auditory memory score of children with DS was significantly lower than that of children in the control group, whereas the visual memory scores of the two groups did not differ. Moreover, children in the control group displayed higher scores for auditory memory than they did for visual memory scores – known as the *modality effect*. Further analysis indicated that the size of the modality effect was 7–18 times greater in the control group than in children with DS. The results of Marcell's three-year study confirmed that individuals with DS showed strong and consistent deficiencies in their ability to recall auditorally presented verbal information.

Table 4.4 summarizes major findings in the studies reviewed above.

Table 4.4 Selected reports on both visual and auditory processing in children with Down's syndrome

| | | |
|---|---|---|
| Bilovsky and Share | 1965 | Input–output circuiting is delayed in auditory–vocal channels and shorter in visual-motor channels |
| Scheffelin | 1968 | Mean error scores in auditory–vocal conditions are twice as large as in visual–motor and visual–vocal conditions |
| Marcell and Armstrong | 1982 | Visual sequential memory is superior to auditory sequential memory |
| Molina and Perez | 1993 | Auditory–verbal modality is weaker than visual–motor modality |
| Marcell | 1994 | Auditory memory scores are lower, but visual memory scores are the same as controls |

## 4.6 Our Investigations of Cognitive and Learning Processes with Focus on Auditory and Visual Sensory Modalities

Since it is assumed that a better understanding of cognitive and learning processes in children with DS may lead to more appropriate educational planning, our studies were designed to investigate both visual and auditory processing in children with this chromosomal disorder using the Kaufman Assessment Battery for Children (1983). The Kaufman test, in particular the mental processing scales, measures the child's ability to solve problems sequentially and simultaneously. Whereas other intelligence tests tend to be more content-oriented, intelligence, as measured with the Kaufman test, is defined in terms of an individual's style of solving problems and processing information.

In our study (Pueschel *et al.* 1987), 20 home-reared children with DS between the ages of 8 and 12½ years, comprised the experimental group. All children had the chromosomal complement of trisomy 21. Their general intellectual functioning was within the mild to moderate range of mental retardation. All children with major medical problems such as severe congenital heart disease and significant sensory impairments including hearing deficits and decreased visual acuity were excluded. All children in the experimental group had early intervention and preschool experiences and were enrolled in an appropriate educational programme.

There were two control groups: one group encompassed 20 younger brothers and sisters of the children with DS. A second control group was formed of non-retarded children who were matched with children of the experimental group according to sex, MA, socioeconomic status of parents and ethnic group.

When we compared the results of sequential processing with simultaneous processing in all three groups, we did not observe any significant difference between the results of the two scales. However, children with DS did poorly in both sequential and simultaneous processing when compared with the two control groups. Follow-up tests indicated that there was a significant difference between the individual groups for both the sequential and the simultaneous processing scale scores. In an analysis of co-variance controlling for MA, the standard scores of sequential and simultaneous processing scales of children with DS were compared with equivalent scores of their brothers and sisters. A significant difference was found for both sequential and simultaneous processing at the $p < 0.001$ level.

In order to investigate whether children with DS performed better in visual processing than in auditory processing, we studied in particular the following subtests of the Kaufman Assessment Battery for Children:

1. *Number Recall*, which uses auditory vocal channels.
2. *Word Order*, which uses auditory-motor channels.
3. *Gestalt Closure,* which uses visual-vocal channels.
4. *Hand Movement,* which uses visual-motor channels.

The results of this analysis indicated that children with DS have significantly more difficulties in their auditory-motor and auditory-vocal channels of communications, They performed significantly less well on the latter two subtests when compared with the subtests which primarily employ visual-motor and visual-vocal channels of communication. When the results of the individual subtests were compared with each other, it was noted that there was a statistically significant difference between Hand Movement and Number Recall, Hand Movement and Word Order, Gestalt Closure and Number Recall, and Gestalt Closure and Word Order. No significant differences were noted contrasting Hand Movement with Gestalt Closure and Number Recall with Word Order.

Since this study as well as previous investigations have found that children with DS ordinarily perform better in visual processing than in auditory processing, one has to question why children with DS show these significant differences and what is the cause of the limited auditory processing in children with DS. Although we lack a basic understanding of the intricate molecular aspects that control these sensory processing events, a developmental–biochemical hypothesis can be advanced in order to explain this phenomenon: myelination of nerve fibres occurs for specific neuronal tissues at different times in the development of the central nervous system. It is well known that nerve fibres of auditory association are myelinated relatively late during neuronal maturation when increased peroxidative damage may occur. Thus, selective perturbation of oxygen-free radical metabolism may adversely affect myelin formation in nerve tracks involved with auditory processing.

Other explanations for the significant auditory processing difficulties in children with DS come from behavioural science research. It has been suggested that children with this chromosome disorder have defective rehearsal mechanisms and impairment of storing information as a result of inadequate language skills. Also, the child's slower encoding at progressively deeper processing levels may be the cause of the reduced auditory processing ability. In addition, short-term memory deficits, storage and retrieval problems, and central auditory processing difficulties may account for the observed results of our studies.

An important aspect of our and other investigations relating to visual and auditory processing in children with DS concerns their psychoeducational implications and educational planning based on the results of various research outcomes. The observed test scores need to be translated into appropriate programmes for effective educational intervention. Since a child's preferred mode of processing information relates closely to the child's learning style and since research supports the notion that effective learning takes place when the mode of teaching matches an individual's preferred processing style, investigations, using the Kaufman test, may provide suggestions that may be effective in teaching specific content. Thus, teaching strategies should capitalize on the children's strengths and should focus primarily on visual-vocal and visual-motor processing modalities in remediation of children with DS. On the other hand, increased emphasis on auditory teaching strategies may potentially lead to frustration for the child and may impede academic progress.

Although it has been demonstrated that it is beneficial for children with a decided strength in one type of processing to be taught by methods that feature these areas, other teaching strategies should, of course, not be excluded in remedial efforts. Built-in flexibility taking into consideration the individual child's strengths and weaknesses should be the central theme of any effective educational programme.

## References


Bilovsky JE and Share J (1965) The ITPA and Down's syndrome: An exploratory study. American Journal of Mental Deficiency 70: 78–82.

Bowler DM, Cufflin J and Kiernan C (1985) Dichotic listening of verbal and nonverbal material by Down's syndrome children and children of normal intelligence. Cortex 21: 637–44.

Catalano RA (1992) Ophthalmologic concerns. In SM Pueschel and JK Pueschel (Eds) Biomedical concerns in persons with Down Syndrome, pp.56–82. Baltimore MD: Brookes.

Dahle AJ and Baldwin RL (1992) Audiologic and otolaryngologic concerns. In SM Pueschel and JK Pueschel (Eds) Biomedical concerns in persons with Down Syndrome, pp.83–107. Baltimore MD: Brookes.

Glenn SM, Cunningham CC and Joyce PF (1981) A study of antibody preferences in nonhandicapped infants and infants with Down's syndrome. Child Development 52: 1303-7.

Gramza AF and Witt PA (1969) Choices of colored blocks in the play of preschool children. Perceptual and Motor Skills 29: 783–7.

Kaufman AS and Kaufman NL (1983) K-ABC Kaufman Assessment Battery for Children. Administration and Scoring Manual. Circle Pines MN: American Guidance Service.

Lincoln AJ, Courchesne E, Kilman BA and Galambos R (1985) Neuropsychological correlates of information-processing by children with Down syndrome. American Journal of Mental Deficiency 89: 403–14.

Marcell MM (1994 April) Auditory and visual digit recall by Down syndrome and other mentally handicapped youth. Paper presented at the International Down Syndrome Conference, Charleston SC.

Marcell MM and Armstrong V (1982) Auditory and visual sequential memory of Down syndrome and nonretarded children. American Journal of Mental Deficiency 87: 86–95.

Marcell MM, Harvey CF and Cothran LP (1988) An attempt to improve auditory short-term memory in Down's syndrome individuals through reducing distractions. Research in Developmental Disabilities 9: 405–17.

Miezejeski CM, Hearney G, Belser R and Sersen EA (1994) Aberrant lateralization of brainstem auditory evoked responses by individuals with Down syndrome. American Journal of Mental Retardation 98: 481–9.

Miranda SB and Fantz RL (1973) Visual preferences of Down's syndrome and normal infants. Child Development 44: 555–61.

Molina S and Perez AA (1993) Cognitive processes in the child with Down syndrome. Developmental Disabilities Bulletin 21: 21–35.

Nakamura H (1965) An inquiry into systematic differences in the abilities of institutionalized adult mongoloids. American Journal of Mental Deficiency 69: 661–5.

Pueschel SM, Gallagher PL, Zartler AS and Pezzullo JC (1987) Cognitive and learning processes in children with Down syndrome. Research in Developmental Disabilities 8: 21–37.

Sackett CP (1967) Response to differentiated visual complexity in four groups of retarded children. Journal of Comparative and Physiological Psychology 64: 200–5.

Salviolo-Negrin N, Soresi S, Baccichetti C, Pozzan G and Trevisan E (1990) Observation on the visual-perceptual abilities and adaptive behavior in adults with Down syndrome. American Journal of Medical Genetics Supplement 7: 309–13.

Scheffelin M (1968) A comparison of four stimulus-response channels in paired-associate learning. American Journal of Mental Deficiency 73: 303–7.

Stratford B (1980) Perception and perceptual-motor processes in children with Down's syndrome. The Journal of Psychology 104: 139–45.

Varnhagen CK, Das JP and Varnhagen S (1987) Auditory and visual memory span: Cognitive processing by TMR individuals with Down syndrome or other etiologies. American Journal of Mental Deficiency 91: 398–405.

Zekulin XY, Gibson D, Mosely JL and Brown RI (1974) Auditory-motor channeling in Down's syndrome subjects. American Journal of Mental Deficiency 78: 571–7.

# 5
# Cross-Domain Relations in Down's Syndrome

**ROBERT M. HODAPP**

## 5.1 Introduction

As opposed to only a few years ago, scientists are now discovering that children vary in their abilities from one domain to another. This issue, called 'cross-domain organization,' has recently challenged workers in a number of areas. Developmental psychologists use cross-domain findings to help inform them about how children's thought is organized, neuropsychologists look for clues to brain organization, and interventionists search for new ways of aiding children's learning. In short, cross-domain organization may be this generation's most important multi-disciplinary topic, an issue that excites researchers and practitioners in a variety of disciplines.

So too with workers in Down's syndrome (DS). In contrast to earlier views that children with DS were simply 'slow' in their development, we are now coming to understand which areas are relative strengths and relative weaknesses for this population. As a result, both research and intervention work is enhanced.

This chapter describes the developmental psychology of cross-domain organization in children with DS. Before discussing such issues, however, it is first important to overview the history of this topic within the larger developmental field. Intellectual profiles for children with DS will then be examined, before the chapter concludes with some remaining issues: the development of children with and without DS; our knowledge of brain organization; and intervention efforts.

## 5.2 How are Developments Organized Across Domains?

Like many topics in developmental psychology, concern over cross-domain organization begins with Jean Piaget. Piaget conceptualized children's intelligence as a series of hierarchically organized stages; he even used the term *structures d'ensemble* to emphasize the horizontal nature of cross-domain organization. To Piaget, the child who is at a specific stage for one type of cognitive functioning is at a similar stage for all areas of cognition. Such horizontally organized stages were even thought to occur within a particular stage. Hence, the infant who is at sensorimotor stage 4 in object permanence is also presumably at sensorimotor stage 4 in means–ends, vocal and gestural imitation, symbolic uses and all other sensorimotor domains.

Figure 5.1 shows this Piagetian, ***structures d'ensemble*** view of horizontally organized stages. As Figure 5.1 demonstrates, the child is at equal or near-equal levels across all domains of functioning. Such a 'flat' or 'even' sense of development has long characterized developmental views toward children with various types of mental retardation (Hodapp and Zigler 1995). Such views have generally led to the idea that children with retardation simply developed 'slower, not differently' than non-retarded children.

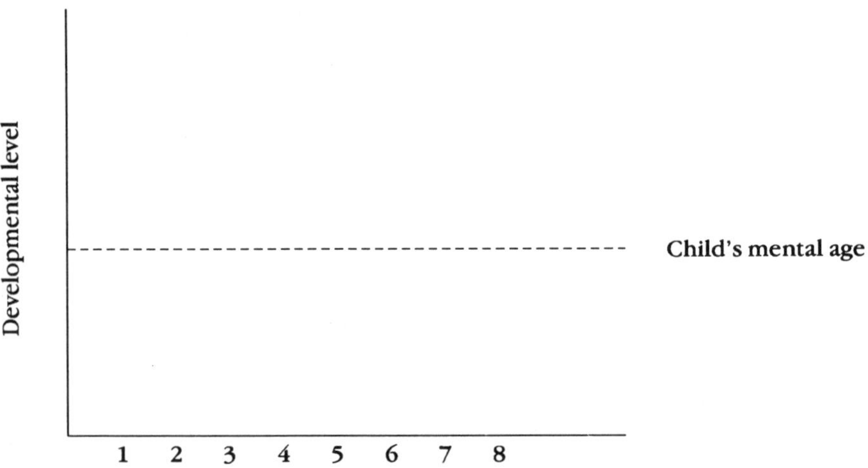


*Figure 5.1* Horizontally organized developmental stages

Although horizontal organization is appealing, such stages have not fared well in recent years. By the early 1980s, Flavell (1982) and Fischer (1980) were suggesting that development was not so perfectly organized from one domain to another, that individual children were often exceptionally high in one area of cognition, but low in another. Fischer (1980) went so far as to suggest that 'unevenness is the rule of development.'

But if a child's levels are not 'in synch' across various domains, what is the organization to development? Two recent suggestions seem important. First, there may be what have been called 'local homologies of shared origin' (Bates *et al.* 1979; Mundy *et al.* 1984). Local homologies are smaller packets of organization; specific skills that do seem to go together in development.

Figure 5.2 shows how local homologies operate. In this figure, we see that clear strengths and weaknesses exist, but at the same time, certain behaviours continue to go together; i.e., there are certain smaller, 'local' areas of horizontal organization. Cicchetti and his colleagues, for example, have found that levels of sensorimotor cognitive abilities correspond closely to types of events eliciting laughter (Cicchetti and Sroufe 1976) and fear (Cicchetti and Sroufe 1978) in children with DS. Similarly, Bates *et al.* (1979) find connections between an infant's levels of means–ends abilities (i.e., use of one object as a means to retrieve another) and early communicative behaviours such as pointing so that the mother can retrieve an object. In several ways, a picture emerges of small areas of organization, but within a larger realm of unevenness.

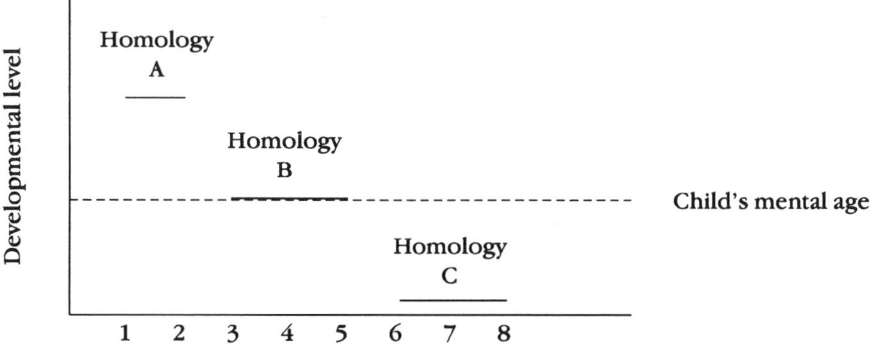


*Figure 5.2* Local homologies in development

There is also a third, slightly different pattern. This idea, from Fodor (1983), is that many different domains may be 'modular,' or 'domain-specific, innately specified, hard-wired, autonomous, and not assembled' (p. 37). Although similar to local homologies, here the emphasis switches to the *differences* in levels of functioning from one domain to another, not on the smaller packets of organization within a domain. One or more individual behaviours may hold together as different systems, but various modules are separated one from another.

The best example of modularity within disabled populations occurs in Williams syndrome (also called infantile hypercalcemia). Williams syndrome is a rare genetic disorder that affects approximately 1 in 20,000 individuals. Resulting from a micro-deletion at the 'elastin gene' on one of the child's two chromosome 7s, Williams syndrome individuals are characterized by 'elfin-lßike' facial features, cardiovascular and renal abnormalities, and moderate to severe levels of mental retardation.

The most striking behavioural feature of Williams syndrome involves these children's high levels of linguistic abilities. As recently noted by Bellugi and her colleagues (Bellugi *et al.* 1994), children with Williams syndrome often show remarkably advanced linguistic abilities, even in the face of lower-level abilities in other areas. Children with overall MA of only about 5 years comprehend words such as 'peninsula' and 'spherical' (Bellugi *et al.* 1988); children with Williams syndrome also demonstrate skills in grammar and storytelling that would seem well beyond their overall mental ages (Reilly *et al.* 1990). Although Udwin and Yule (1990) have recently questioned whether all children with Williams syndrome show this profile of 'language in the (relative) absence of thought,' many do.

In addition to many children with Williams syndrome, several exceptional individual cases show unusual profiles of abilities. Most prominent among these extraordinary individuals is Genie – the young woman studied by Curtiss (1976) who was rescued after having lived the first 14 years of her life in almost total neglect. In the years after her rescue, Genie developed an extensive vocabulary and an array of pragmatic skills, but was never quite able to acquire English grammar. Conversely, Yamada (1990) describes a young woman named Laura, who, like children with Williams syndrome, showed remarkably advanced linguistic abilities in the face of very low overall functioning (see also Rondal, Chapter 7). In both Williams syndrome and these exceptional individual cases, different domains seem to develop separately, one from another. This idea of modularity pervades much recent thinking in developmental psychology.

## 5.3 Cross-Domain Relations in Down's Syndrome

Turning to Down's syndrome, we see that many different areas of deficit have been considered characteristic of this disorder. But before addressing this issue, two preliminary points need to be addressed.

### 5.3.1 Preliminary issues

First, the studies described below examine only children with DS, not children with 'mental retardation,' or 'organic impairments' or 'mixed groups.' Given this book's exclusive focus on Down's syndrome, it is especially surprising how rarely behavioural researchers examine children with specific etiologies of mental retardation. As Hodapp and Dykens (1994) noted, few behavioural studies exist on many different etiologies of mental retardation. Down's syndrome alone, it seems, is an exception to this rule. Across the many journals surveyed over the period 1985–1990, 73 behavioural studies appeared on DS, as compared with only 40 on fragile X syndrome, seven on Prader-Willi syndrome, eight on Rett syndrome, three on Turner syndrome, and five on Williams syndrome.

In considering this state of affairs, Hodapp and Dykens (1994) describe what they call the 'two cultures' of behavioural work in mental retardation. As seen in Table 5.1, one can distinguish between 'level-of-impairment' and 'etiology-based' researchers. Level-of-impairment researchers generally form their research groups on the basis of the individual's level of impairment: the mild, moderate, severe and profound levels that have historically characterized mental retardation work. These researchers show less regard for the cause of the child's retardation. Many psychologists and special educators are level-of-impairment workers. In contrast, etiology-based workers form their research groups based on the child's type of mental retardation. The child's level of impairment receives less emphasis. Geneticists, child psychiatrists, pediatricians and other, predominantly medically-oriented workers adhere to etiology-based approaches to studying behavioural functioning in mental retardation.

As Table 5.1 also notes, both perspectives have their strengths and weaknesses. By being unconcerned about the child's etiology of mental retardation, level-of-impairment workers often do not appreciate important genetic and other advances. Conversely, etiology-based researchers are often less well-versed in behavioural work. Thus, while etiology-based researchers generally examine IQ and gross aspects of behavioural functioning, other, more sophisticated work is rarely performed. Hence, particularly in those syndromes for which little work has been performed (Prader-Willi, Rett, etc.), even less work has examined sophisticated issues of language, cognitive or social development, or information-processing, psychopathology, families or specific interventions.

As a result, we often do not know the extent to which any strengths or weaknesses found in DS or other groups are 'etiology-specific' or true of

Table 5.1 Characteristics of the two cultures of behavioural research in mental retardation

| Level-of-impairment-Based | Etiology-based |
|---|---|
| Main characteristics | |
| Group by degree of disability | Group by etiology |
| Less regard for genetic etiology | De-emphasize degree of disability |
| Professions (with some overlap) | |
| Behavioural psychologists | Geneticists |
| Special educators | Genetic counsellors |
| Clinical psychologists | Child psychiatrists |
| Social workers | Pediatricians |
| | Psychiatrists |
| Strengths | |
| Advances in behavioural measurement | Advances in molecular genetics |
| Weaknesses | |
| Often less aware of advances in genetics and molecular genetics | Often less sophisticated in behavioural measurement |
| Often less appreciation for impact of genetic etiology on research | Often less application of findings to pertinent issues or intervention in larger mental retardation field |

all children with mental retardation. We are also often unable to characterize individual differences within a syndrome, or why such individual differences might occur. Most importantly, we are unable to learn specific information about development, brain-behaviour relations or strategies of intervention.

A second preliminary issue concerns the definition of a 'weakness' and of a 'strength'. All of the studies described below compare the child's behaviour in one specific area of development with overall mental age (MA) or other 'level-of-functioning' measures. This comparison may work in one of two ways. First, weaknesses and strengths may be examined within individual children with DS. Thus, one can compare the child's level of language to that same child's overall MA. Or, alternatively, strengths and weaknesses may be examined by comparing language levels of groups of children with DS to MA-matched non-retarded children. Either way, the resulting strength or weakness is a relative strength or weakness, i.e., a strength or weakness compared with the child's overall abilities.

While the point may seem obvious, it is one that is too often overlooked. If one wants to know whether individuals with DS show a relative strength or weakness in a specific area of functioning, one must compare functioning in the domain of interest to overall MA, mean length of utterance (MLU), or other 'level-of-functioning' measures. Comparisons to children of the same chronological age (CA) – which are those most often performed in the mental retardation field – will not suffice. As Cicchetti and Pogge-Hesse (1982) note in criticizing studies that compare children with DS with non-retarded children of the same CA instead of MA: *'We know that they are retarded; the important and challenging research questions concern the developmental process'* (p. 279). The studies described below compare functioning in children with DS to MA or other level-of-functioning measures.

### 5.3.2 Findings of strengths–weaknesses

Once compared to such level-of-functioning measures, what do we find? First, that children with DS do not show extreme strengths and weaknesses on every measure.

Compare, for example, functioning on various domains of the Kaufman Assessment Battery for Children (K-ABC) (Kaufman and Kaufman 1983). The K-ABC is a psychometric instrument for children aged 2 ½–12 years. In contrast to other IQ tests, the K-ABC is specifically tied to two types of mental functioning – sequential processing and simultaneous processing. Sequential processing involves the solving of problems in serial or temporal order. Subtests in this domain require children to repeat a series of hand movements performed by the examiner, or repeat a series of numbers, or to point to a set of pictures first named by the examiner. In contrast, simultaneous processing involves the integration of stimuli in a holistic, Gestalt-like manner. Subtests in this domain involve such things as recognizing a drawing when provided with only parts of several lines, arranging triangles to make a design, or in other ways understanding the whole picture.

In work with children with DS, Hodapp *et al.* (1993) and Pueschel *et al.* (1987) have shown that these children are reasonably even from one domain to another on the major domains of the K-ABC. That is, these children show levels in sequential, or bit-by-bit serial, processing, that are similar to their levels on simultaneous, or holistic, processing. Children with DS, then, do not differ from MA-matches on at least certain intellectual tasks. Compared with the findings from such disorders as Williams syndrome, the peaks and valleys of Down's syndrome may not be quite as striking.

Yet, when examined more closely, children with this disorder do show certain areas of strength and weakness. Table 5.2 reviews some of these hypothesized strengths and weaknesses. Clearly, a greater number of weaknesses than strengths have been proposed over the years, and the list of weaknesses is very long. Candidates for weaknesses include language, speech, auditory sequential processing, maths, attention, arousal and many other areas.

Across these areas, however, a few things stand out. Most prominently, many of the hypothesized weaknesses appear in language. The grammar findings of Fowler, Rondal, and Miller (see below), Miller's finding of 'receptive over expressive language' and Miller's findings of expressive language levels below overall MA are all evidence that language is a

Table 5.2 Proposed areas of strengths and weaknesses in Down's syndrome

| | |
|---|---|
| *Proposed weaknesses* | |
| language | mathematics |
| expressive language | abstract symbol systems |
| grammar | visually directed reaching |
| articulation | visual monitoring |
| auditory processing | hypotonia |
| non-verbal requesting behaviours | low reactivity |
| low task persistence | slow orienting to auditory information |
| inadequate motor organization | inadequate cerebral specialization |
| *Proposed strengths* | |
| social skills | adaptive behaviour |
| most non-verbal social interaction skills | pleasant personality |
| protection from some forms of psychopathology (e.g., bipolar depression and psychoses) | |

relative weakness for these children. At first glance, it appears that language is an area of particular difficulty for children with DS.

On the opposite side, social skills – and possibly 'pleasant personalities and relative freedom from at least some forms of psychopathology' (Dykens 1995) – seem to be relative strengths. Even during the early years, these children appear to show strengths in non-verbal social interaction skills – such things as reaching toward, making eye contact with, playing with, or taking interactive turns with an adult experimenter (Mundy *et al.* 1988). This overall picture – of weaknesses in language and strengths in social skills – seems agreed-upon by most professionals working with children with DS.

Table 5.3 further illustrates this issue by focusing on four studies, two of grammar and two of social-adaptive skills. These studies have been chosen to make three points that are central to any discussion of the developmental aspects of cross-domain organization. Specifically, the three points are:

- that strengths and weaknesses are not static over development;
- that development and cross-domain relations are therefore related;
- and that we are only just beginning to understand what constitutes a 'domain' of functioning.

First, Table 5.3 indicates that ***strengths and weaknesses may not be static***, but instead change with development. The best example here is Miller's (1992) findings of changing numbers of children who show the

Table 5.3 Developmental aspects of strengths and weaknesses in Down's syndrome

| Study | Profile | Specific findings |
|---|---|---|
| **A:** Grammar | | |
| Fowler 1994 | weakness in grammar | slowdown at Brown's Stage III most aspects of grammar similarly impaired |
| Miller 1992 | expressive language deficits (compared with receptive language and MA) | more subjects show expressive deficits with increasing MA |
| **B:** Social-adaptive skills | | |
| Mundy, *et al.* 1988 | Strength (compared with MA matches) on most non-verbal social interaction skills | strengths in most skills, but weakness in non-verbal behaviours |
| Tingey, *et al.* 1991 | slowed development in many areas over first 6 years slowed than personal and | communication and cognitive domains more than social domains |

pattern of receptive over expressive language, or of language below MA levels. Receptive skills may exceed skills in expressive language for some children early on, but more and more children exhibit this discrepancy (to increasingly greater degrees) as the child develops in language.

In a similar way, note Fowler's (1988) findings concerning the development of grammar. Although studied both cross-sectionally and longitudinally with small groups, Fowler finds that abilities in grammar seem to increase with increasing chronological age until the child approaches Brown's MLU Stage III, but not much thereafter. Brown's Stage III is an interesting moment in grammatical development. This stage is defined by average sentence lengths of 2.50–3.25 morphemes per utterance; typically developing children usually go through this stage from the ages of 30–36 months. Already having mastered most of the basic meaning relations, during Stage III the child begins developing such complex syntactic structures as negatives, wh-questions, and yes-no questions. In many ways, Stage III is the first of the 'truly grammatical' stages in language development (the earlier stages being characterized by basic word order and case relations).

On reaching Stage III language, grammar becomes increasingly challenging for children with DS. From this point forward, young children with DS have tremendous difficulty. A study by Rondal *et al.* (1988) shows this difficulty clearly. Correlating Brown's first three Stages of language development and chronological ages in children with DS, Rondal *et al.* (1988) found an overall correlation of 0.87. However, this correlation varies widely depending on which level of language one is considering. At earlier levels of grammar, correlations are extremely high between the child's CA and MLU: during these early stages of language, the older the child, the higher the MLU. However, no correlation exists between MLU and CA for children whose MLUs are above 2.00 (2.00–3.50): this correlation is almost exactly zero ($r = -0.004$). Thus, the straightforward relation between increasing age and increasing grammar ceases as many children with DS become 'stuck' in their development of grammar.

A second, similar point is that ***development and cross-domain organization are related***. If Brown's Stage III of grammar is particularly problematic – if at this point many children with DS find it difficult to advance in grammar – then an already weak area of development becomes relatively weaker. We might, then, be better off changing our thinking slightly. Instead of thinking about 'grammar as a weakness' for children with DS, we might consider 'grammar as a weakness once a certain level of grammatical ability is acquired.'

Consider Miller's (1988, 1992) work as another example of intellectual profiles that shift with development. As noted in Table 5.2, expressive language is delayed over receptive language in children with DS. Examined more closely, however, Miller too finds a shift with development. Whereas productive language ages and mental ages are often about even when the child's MA is below 24 months, discrepancies become increasingly apparent later. Thus, whereas 54%–61% of children (depending on the testing session) showed productive language deficits when MAs were 24 months or below, 83%–100% of subjects with MAs above 25 months showed productive deficits. Again, we have an emerging weakness, a domain that, with development, becomes relatively weaker in individual children (and that shows itself as a weakness for more and more children). Thus, one cannot examine cross-domain relations in children without simultaneously examining how such interrelations change as the child develops.

The third issue concerns the ***nature of domains of development***. We are accustomed to thinking of language, social skills, cognitive skills and motor skills as 'domains of development'. We are further accustomed to dividing these areas into smaller sub-areas, topic areas that we assume do indeed hold together in terms of the child's development. At present, we do not exactly know what constitutes a domain of functioning. For example, should language be considered as a single entity, or should language skills themselves be divided? (See Rondal, Chapter 7, for further discussions of this issue.) Similarly, are intellectual abilities all one thing, or do we have seven different intelligences as Gardner (1983) suggests? Or, examined another way, should we conceptualize domains as various all-purpose skills that cut across content areas? Some all-purpose skills that may cross content areas include sequential or simultaneous processing, and expressive versus receptive abilities. What, in short, is the best way to conceptualize intelligence? For now, we cannot say for certain.

There are, however, certain clues, some of which have arisen from work with retarded populations, some from Down's syndrome. From studies of individual cases like Laura and Genie, and from studies of Williams syndrome, grammar seems to hold together as a separate skill. Similarly, in work with children with DS, grammar also holds together as a separate skill, at least at specific points during development. For example, children with DS score at almost the identical levels in grammar when MLU measures are compared with other grammar measures, such as Scarborough's new Index of Productive Syntax (IPSyn) measure (Scarborough *et al.* 1991).

More to the point, different sub-areas of grammar seem to develop at equal or near-equal levels. In the most careful and detailed work to date, both Rondal and Fowler find that, when matched to non-retarded children on levels of grammar – as measured by the MLU – children with DS do not differ from non-retarded children on most grammatical features. For example, Rondal (1987) has found that, when matched on MLU to non-retarded children, children with DS are similar in their amounts of utterances without a verb, or on declaratives, imperatives, wh-questions and yes-no questions. Fowler *et al.* (1994) find similarities between DS and typically developing, MLU-matched children in noun phrases, verbs per utterance, conjunctions, negatives, passives, possessive forms, and almost all other aspects of grammar. As in children with other forms of mental retardation, children with DS also appear to have a grammatical system that is coherent, systematic and modular. These children may have great difficulty acquiring that grammatical system, but it seems a coherent system nonetheless.

In contrast, early social and adaptive skills may not go together as a single entity. As shown in Table 5.3, Mundy *et al.* (1988) find that, whereas children with DS show a relative strength in some aspects of social skills, their non-verbal requesting abilities are below MA-levels – and as non-verbal requesting abilities may relate to expressive language levels, this differentiation of early social skills may be important. In essence, while grammar seems a single entity after the 2- or 3-year level, early social skills may need to be considered on a more individual basis.

In addition, adaptive behaviour may not hold together as clearly as one single entity. As Tingey *et al.* (1991) show, certain adaptive domains slow more than others in the early development of children with DS. Specifically, those adaptive domains that seem most cognitive and linguistic slow more than those which are more personal and social. This study shows that one cannot take, at face value, the various domains of functioning from different intellectual or adaptive scales.

To recapitulate, children with DS do appear to show particular strengths and weaknesses. So far, the best candidates for strengths appear to be various aspects of social skills; various linguistic abilities seem the most likely weaknesses. But even within such strengths and weaknesses, we need to consider issues such as the exact set of skills that should be considered a strength or weakness, and the changes that occur with development.

## 5.4 Applications

Three applications of these findings seem apparent. Although none of these areas is as yet well-examined, all promise to develop in coming years.

### 5.4.1 Knowledge of cross-domain relations

As previously noted, we do not know exactly which aspects of development hang together. The first application thus concerns increasing knowledge of cross-domain relations. For example, future years promise to tell us if indeed grammar is its own separable entity, or, if not, how grammar fits within a larger domain of language. Similarly, researchers should, over the next few years, determine the degree to which 'all-purpose' strategies (e.g., sequential *v.s* simultaneous processing) cut across content areas, as well as determining the effects of having particular strengths and weaknesses.

Such knowledge is central to our understanding of typically developing children, children with other retardation conditions, and, ultimately, for children with DS. Indeed, there seems an interplay between typical and atypical development. Increasingly, we use our knowledge of development in retardation to tell us about typical development, and vice-versa (Hodapp and Burack 1990). In future years, we can expect such cross-fertilization to increase our knowledge of both typical development and of development in various mental retardation syndromes, including Down's syndrome.

### 5.4.2 Knowledge about brain involvement and development

A second outgrowth of cross-domain work concerns the brain. Just as work on cross-domain relations is relatively recent – and is only beginning to tell us how developments go together – so too are neuropsychology and developmental neuropsychology relatively new fields. We are only beginning to link changes in brain development with behavioural advances. To give what may be the best example, Fischer (1987) has taken Diamond's (1987) work on delayed imitation and short-term memory in primates and tied these changes to specific developments in sensorimotor functioning in the human infant. Granted, all of this work is preliminary. Yet over the next decade, we will know more about how the brain develops and how such neurological development underlies specific cognitive developments and cross-domain relations.

### 5.4.3 Knowledge about intervention

Ultimately, all of our knowledge aims at understanding how to help children with DS and other forms of mental retardation. Thus, intervention is the third application of our burgeoning knowledge of cross-domain relations.

Partly because of the two cultures of mental retardation, we do not yet have such a targeted, specific intervention for children with DS. Instead, most intervention programmes are 'generic' rather than 'etiology-based.' Yet as we learn more about specific areas of strengths and weaknesses in DS, and about how such intellectual profiles change with development, we are increasingly in the position to offer this, more specific, 'Down's syndrome intervention.' This intervention might capitalize on training grammatical morphemes, if this is indeed the main problem in the language of these children. Conversely, if the ultimate problem is found to be sequential processing or some other ability that cuts across various domains, then this too might be open to intervention.

Various workers have now called for such etiology-based interventions (Gibson 1991; Hodapp and Dykens 1991). In different ways, all have argued for the specialness of Down's syndrome, of fragile X syndrome, and of many different mental retardation conditions. Although granting that each disorder will not be unique on everything – and that individual differences exist within each syndrome – such workers nevertheless hold that interventions informed by the child's etiology will be better, more specifically targeted, and, ultimately, more effective.

But, at least in the United States, etiology-based interventions have often met with resistance. Most workers do not see the benefits of an etiology-based approach. Some (e.g., Forness 1993) fear the 'Balkanization' of special education services, with every different type of retardation requiring its own specialized services. The fear is that mainstreaming and the integration of children with retardation will be hampered if each requires a separate, etiology-specific programme of intervention. But while appreciating the problems inherent in etiology-based interventions, such difficulties may have been over-sold. After all, what is an 'Individualized Educational Plan' (IEP) for a child with DS if it does not capitalize on the syndrome's specific strengths and weaknesses? How can one justify special educational services for these children which do not consider that DS may differ from other retardation disorders?

In all these areas, we currently have more questions than answers. The answers involve studies showing that, in DS, a specific intellectual profile seems to be emerging, and that this profile becomes more pronounced over time. Furthermore, this profile – particularly its suggestions about grammar as a modular system – complements recent work on other syndromes and on exceptional individuals such as Genie and Laura. The remaining questions involve specifying the exact nature of a domain of functioning, the exact strengths and weaknesses in DS, and the exact applications to both our research and our interventions. Although this chapter presents many more questions than answers, my hope is that it stimulates further work concerning the cross-domain organization of intelligence – and how this changes with development – in children with DS.

## References

Bates E, Benigni L, Bretherton I, Camaioni L and Volterra V (1979) The emergence of symbols: Cognition and communication in infancy. New York: Academic Press.

Bellugi U, Marks S, Bihrle A and Sabo H (1988) Dissociation between language and cognitive functions in Williams syndrome. In D Bishop and K Mogford (Eds) Language development in exceptional circumstances, pp.177–89. London: Churchill Livingstone.

Bellugi U, Wang P and Jerrigan T (1994) Williams Syndrome: An unusual neuropsychological profile. In SH Broman and J Grafman (Eds) Atypical cognitive deficits in developmental disorders, pp.23–56. Hillsdale NJ: Erlbaum

Cicchetti D and Pogge-Hesse P (1982) Possible contributions of the study of organically retarded persons to developmental theory. In E Zigler and D Balla (Eds) Mental retardation: The developmental-difference controversy, pp.277–318. Hillsdale NJ: Erlbaum.

Cicchetti D and Sroufe LA (1976) The relationship between affective and cognitive development in Down syndrome infants. Child Development 47: 290–2.

Cicchetti D and Sroufe LA (1978) An organizational view of affect: Illustration from the study of Down syndrome infants. In M Lewis and LA Rosenblum (Eds) The development of affect, pp.29–38. New York: Plenum.

Curtiss S (1976) Genie: The story of a modern day 'wild child'. New York: Academic Press.

Diamond A (1987) Development of the ability to use recall to guide action, as indicated by infants' performance on AB. Child Development 56: 868–83.

Dykens EM (1995) (in press) DNA meets DSM: Genetic syndromes growing importance in dual diagnosis. Mental Retardation.

Fischer K (1980) A theory of cognitive development: The control and construction of a hierarchy of skills. Psychological Review 87: 477–531.

Fischer K (1987) Relations between brain and cognitive development. Child Development 58: 623–32.

Flavell J (1982) Structures, stages, and sequences in cognitive development. In WA Collins (Ed) The concept of development: The Minnesota Symposia on Child Psychology 15: 1–27. Hillsdale, NJ: Erlbaum.

Fodor J (1983) Modularity of mind: An essay on faculty psychology. Cambridge MA: MIT Press.

Forness SR (1993) The Balkanization of Special Education: Proliferation and categories and sub-categories for 'new' disorders. In J Marr, G Sugai and G Tindal (Eds) The Oregon Conference Monograph 5: 117–32. Eugene OR: University of Oregon.

Fowler A (1988) Determinants of rate of language growth in children with Down Syndrome. In L Nadel (Ed) The psychobiology of Down Syndrome, pp.217–45. Cambridge MA: MIT Press.

Fowler A (1990) Language abilities in children with Down Syndrome: Evidence for a specific syntactic delay. In D Cicchetti and M Beeghly (Eds) Children with Down Syndrome: A developmental approach, pp.302–28. New York: Cambridge University Press.

Fowler A, Gelman R and Gleitman L (1994) The course of language learning in children with Down Syndrome. In H Tager-Flusberg (Ed) Constraints on language acquisition: Studies of atypical children, pp.91–140. Hillsdale NJ: Erlbaum.

Gardner H (1983) Frames of mind. New York: Basic Books.

Gibson D (1991) Down syndrome and cognitive enhancement: Not like the others. In K Marfo (Ed) Early intervention in transition: Current perspectives on programs for handicapped children, pp.61–90. New York: Praeger.

Hodapp RM and Burack JA (1990) What mental retardation tells us about typical development: The examples of sequences, rates, and cross-domain relations. Development and Psychopathology 2: 213–26.

Hodapp RM and Dykens EM (1991) Toward an etiology-specific strategy of early intervention with handicapped children. In K Marfo (Ed) Early intervention in transition: Current perspectives on programs for handicapped children, pp.41–60. New York: Praeger.

Hodapp RM and Dykens EM (1994) Mental retardation's two cultures of behavioral research. American Journal on Mental Retardation 98: 675–87.

Hodapp RM, Leckman JF, Dykens EM, Sparrow S, Zelinsky D and Ort SI (1993) K-ABC profiles in children with fragile X syndrome, Down syndrome, and nonspecific mental retardation. American Journal on Mental Retardation 97: 39–46.

Hodapp RM and Zigler E (1995) Past, present, and future issues in the developmental approach to mental retardation and developmental disabilities. In D Cicchetti and D Cohen (Eds) Developmental psychopathology Vol.2. Risk, disorder, and adaptation, pp.299–331. New York: Wiley.

Kaufman AS and Kaufman NL (1983) Kaufman Assessment Battery for Children. Circle Pines MN: American Guidance Service.

Miller J (1988) The developmental asynchrony of language development in children with Down Syndrome. In L Nadel (Ed) The psychobiology of Down Syndrome, pp.167–98. Cambridge MA: MIT Press.

Miller J (1992) Lexical development in young children with Down Syndrome. In R Chapman (Ed) Processes in language acquisition and disorders, pp.202–16. St. Louis MO: Mosby.

Mundy P, Siebert J and Hogan A (1984) Relationship between sensorimotor and early communication abilities in developmentally delayed children. Merrill-Palmer Quarterly 30: 33–48.

Mundy P, Sigman M, Kasari C and Yirmiya N (1988) Nonverbal communication skills in Down syndrome children. Child Development 59: 235–49.

Pueschel S, Gallagher P, Zartler A and Pezzullo J (1987) Cognitive and learning processes in children with Down Syndrome. Research in Developmental Disabilities 8: 21–37.

Reilly JS, Klima E and Bellugi U (1990) Once more with feeling: Affect and language in atypical populations. Development and Psychopathology 2: 367–91.

Rondal JA (1987) Language development and mental retardation. In W Yule and M Rutter (Eds) Language development and disorders. Clinics in Developmental Medicine 101/102: 248–61. Oxford: MacKeith Press.

Rondal JA, Ghiotto M, Brédart S and Bachelet J-F (1988) Mean length of utterance of children with Down Syndrome. American Journal on Mental Retardation 93: 64–6.

Scarborough H, Rescorla L, Tager-Flusberg H, Fowler A and Sudhalter V (1991) The relation of utterance length to grammatical complexity in normal and language-disabled groups. Applied Psycholinguistics 12: 23–45.

Tager-Flusberg H (1994) Contributions to the field of language acquisition from research on atypical children. In H Tager-Flusberg (Ed) Constraints on language acquisition: Studies of atypical children, pp.1–8. Hillsdale NJ: Erlbaum.

Tingey C, Mortensen L, Matheson P and Doret W (1991) Developmental attainments of infants and young children with Down syndrome. International Journal of Disability, Development and Education 38: 15–26.

Udwin O and Yule W (1990) Expressive language of children with Williams Syndrome. American Journal of Medical Genetics Supplement 6: 108–14.

Yamada JE (1990) Laura: A case for the modularity of language. Cambridge MA: MIT Press.

# 6
# Learning in Young Children with Down's Syndrome: Developmental Trends

JENNIFER G WISHART

## 6.1 Introduction

This chapter looks at how young children with Down's syndrome (DS) approach the task of learning. It addresses the question of whether a specific 'style' of learning is associated with the syndrome and if so, whether this changes as the children grow older and their experience of learning increases. In our own research we have looked in particular at whether children with DS may be *adding* to their already-existing difficulties by making inefficient use of their skills and using avoidance strategies when presented with opportunities for learning new skills. Our longitudinal data suggest that with increasing age, the children often change from being active and relatively able problem-solvers into progressively more reluctant learners. Deficits in their motivation to learn would appear to be significantly undermining their progress, not only delaying the acquisition and consolidation of new skills but also denying them the full benefits of skills they already have.

Surprisingly little attention is currently being paid to the contribution of motivational deficits to learning difficulties in children with DS, or indeed to the role of psychological factors in general in determining developmental outcome. Despite the very large numbers of children affected by the syndrome and the intrinsic interest of DS itself, only a very small number of psychologists are investigating how the condition directly affects behavioural development. In comparison with the attention directed at DS by the biological sciences, psychological research on the syndrome is very thin on the ground indeed. Children with DS are much more likely to be used as control children in studies of normal cognitive development than studied in their own right and as a result, we are still a disappointingly long way from understanding the exact nature of their learning difficulties. Until we can improve on present levels of knowledge, our ability to help the children to compensate for their difficulties remains severely limited.

## 6.2 Earlier Work on Cognitive Development in DS

It is over a century since Langdon Down first described DS and between then and now there have been a great many studies of cognitive ability in children with DS (for overviews, see Gibson 1978; Cicchetti and Beeghly 1990). Some highly revealing research – with findings still useful today – was carried out during this time but unfortunately much of this earlier body of work on DS now has little relevance because most of the children in studies carried out prior to the 60s were being raised in institutions. And if there is one psychological fact that is almost universally accepted, it is that institutional life does nothing for the development and maintenance of cognitive skills – in anyone, with or without DS.

By the late 60s/early 70s, the majority of children with DS were being brought up by their parents in the family home. Here too, though, there are problems with many of the studies carried out, albeit of a quite different kind. Attitudes towards DS were much more enlightened by this time and a great deal of research carried out in these years undoubtedly had the very best interests of the children at heart. In their enthusiasm to help, however, many studies regrettably paid insufficient attention to the rudimentary rules of scientific enquiry. As a result, some of their findings are at best very difficult to evaluate, and at worst, potentially highly misleading.

Early intervention studies from this period are perhaps the worst culprits in this respect. Many of the first, ground-breaking programmes claimed very high success rates in raising achievement levels in young children with DS. The majority, however, assessed success only by comparing the progress of children in their programme against available developmental norms for children with DS. These norms were typically drawn from children almost all of whom would have been institutionalized from birth; little use was made of concurrent control groups of children who were living at home but not receiving early intervention. It would have been very surprising indeed if *any* group of children with DS being brought up at home in the 70s and 80s had not exceeded norms from institutionalized children of the 50s and 60s, regardless of whether they were receiving early intervention or not. This, it must be remembered, was a time when interest in early child development was at a peak, when the importance of the mother–child relationship was exalted to its highest-ever level, and which saw the emergence of a completely new industry – *educational toys*. Early stimulation was seen by many as holding the key to enhancing intelligence levels – both in children with and without learning disabilities – and this increase in learning opportunities was soon reflected in earlier ages of acquisition of many developmental milestones.

Objectively evaluating the efficacy of these first early intervention programmes was in any case virtually impossible. Many programmes involved only very small numbers of children and were often under constant revision during the period of intervention. Basic features of the intervention – such as age of the child at entry; length of participation in the programme; frequency and content of sessions; level of input expected from parents – were often poorly controlled and varied greatly from programme to programme. Those who designed and implemented the programmes often reported major gains in the young children with DS receiving early intervention, but independent reviewers were generally far less impressed by the measurable levels of success achieved by most programmes (see Hayden and Dmitriev 1975; Spitz 1986; Gibson and Harris 1988). Many gains proved to have very poor 'tenacity' and therefore had little true developmental value. Any advantage proved to be very short-lived and children not being given any specific training soon caught up (Sloper *et al.* 1986).

The widespread availability of early intervention programmes is often given the credit for the higher levels of competence which today's young children with DS show. To a great many researchers, however, it seems just as likely that these advances stem from the better management of the children's health problems, the more positive attitudes of their parents and teachers, and their greatly increased access to education and a more normal lifestyle. There is indeed some concern amongst professionals that an uncritical belief in the direct efficacy of early intervention may lead people to underestimate the degree of learning difficulties likely to show up in post-infancy years and to persist throughout childhood and into adult years.

## 6.3 Cognitive Abilities in Children with DS

Children with DS show enormous individual variability in the ages at which specific cognitive milestones are reached and in the levels of cognitive achievement ultimately reached (Cunningham 1987). However, it is important that people recognize the problems that nearly all of them face in learning even very basic childhood skills. Many children with DS do not progress much beyond the intellectual capabilities of the average 6–8 year old and a significant number do not achieve even that; mastering language skills, whether spoken or written, also remains a major problem for a great many (see Rondal, in Chapter 7 of this volume).

Cognitive skills, along with language skills, have thus far proved very resistant to attempts at facilitative intervention but lack of success to date does not imply that we should give up on our efforts. There are considerable grounds for believing that with a better understanding of the very *specific* nature of the learning difficulties experienced by children with DS, much more effective methods of intervening may still be found. The emphasis here is very much on the word 'specific'. The specific nature of these difficulties is likely to demand a major change in our approach to teaching children with DS, one which recognizes, for example, their short-term memory problems, their deficits in auditory and visual sequential memory, and the relative strength of visual over their auditory processing ability (Marcell and Armstrong 1982; Varnhagen *et al.* 1987; Bower and Hayes 1994). Current models of educational intervention do not recognize the specific educational needs of children with DS adequately, and some make incorrect assumptions about how development proceeds in DS. This may well be why we have seen much less progress than we might have hoped for to date, especially in older children (see Buckley, in Chapter 8 of this volume).

## 6.4 The Nature of Cognitive Development in DS

It is widely assumed, implicitly if not always explicitly, that cognitive development in children with DS can basically be understood in terms of a slowed-down version of normal development: that it is only the rate and endpoint that distinguishes their development from that of other children. This seems unlikely to be an accurate characterization of the nature of development in DS. It seems far more likely that there are significant and very important differences in how development unfolds in children with DS, some of these stemming as much from crucial differences in the psychological environment in which they learn as from the biological disadvantages they carry from birth.

Maintaining that development in children with DS is fundamentally different may not be the favoured viewpoint but it does fit with the large body of data from the neurosciences showing major differences in the structure of the DS brain and in how it works (Uecker *et al.* 1993). It is clear that children with DS are at a considerable disadvantage when it comes to the basic tools for learning. This inherent biological disadvantage can only be compounded by the adverse psychological effects of always being in the 'slow lane' when it comes to learning. For most children with DS, progress in virtually all developmental domains is likely to take much longer, failure is more frequent, and the expectations of those around them, whether parents or professionals, are typically low. All of this must make learning a very different experience for the child with DS. Provided with a far-from-perfect set of tools for learning and with a very different psychological environment in which to learn, it would surely be remarkable if development in DS children did *not* follow different pathways to those seen in normally-developing children from a very early stage.

## 6.5 Increasing Age, Increasing Problems ?

One of the more robust findings about cognitive development in DS is that IQ level typically declines with increasing age. Carr (1985) reviewed a large number of IQ studies carried out between 1961–1982, looking at data from over 2500 children who had been tested at varying intervals and at various ages between birth and 18 years. She found evidence of a steep drop in IQ between 1 and 3 years, with this decline continuing, through to age 13 (the highest age level for which there was sufficient data to plot developmental trends), although lessening in slope. The same pattern also emerged in a recent cross-sectional study of 35 children with DS aged 3 months to 5 years we ourselves tested, despite the fact that all of our children had been receiving early intervention in the form of regular visits from an educational home visitor (Duffy 1990; Wishart, in press).

One of the main aims of our research programme has therefore been to try to pinpoint some of the factors underlying this failure to maintain developmental rate. The following is a brief overview of some of our findings along with some illustrative data. The children with DS in our studies have ranged in age from birth to 14 years. In longitudinal studies data collection has extended from 1 to 5 years, depending on the age of subjects at entry and the nature of the study in question. In all of the studies, control groups of children without DS have been included to allow direct evaluation of difference versus delay theories of development. Typically, normally-developing (ND) children were matched with the children with DS for either chronological age (CA) or for stage in development, depending on the focus of the particular study. As will be apparent from some of the findings, however, 'matching' is a somewhat misleading and sometimes meaningless concept when it comes to DS. Children with DS simply do not respond in test situations in the same way as ND children, even when they achieve similar 'scores'. Children with DS do not even provide satisfactory matches for themselves at times: often, their responses on a given test fluctuate greatly over two identical, closely-spaced testing sessions, with successes in the first session no longer demonstrated in the second session and 'failures' turning into successes.

Findings from the three sets of studies to be outlined below – on operant learning, object concept development, and IQ tests – all demonstrate some of the key features which would appear to define early development in DS: the growing use of avoidance strategies when faced with cognitive challenges; the less-than-efficient use of existing problem-solving skills; the failure to consolidate newly-acquired cognitive skills into the repertoire, and the increasing reluctance to take the initiative in learning.

## 6.6 Developmental Trends in Operant Learning

Our studies of operant learning provide the most direct evidence that young children with DS very quickly learn to depend on the support of others in learning contexts, even when that support is not needed. Operant learning studies investigate the ability of children to detect that their activity had caused something to happen. Understanding this kind of relationship is basic to learning and is also essential to the formation of any belief in self-efficacy – that you have some control over what happens around you and to you.

Fifty infants with DS between birth and two years of age took part in cross-sectional and longitudinal studies (Wishart 1990, 1991, 1993a). Because children with DS often have poor muscle tone in the early years, a task suitable for use with the youngest and least motorically-able children was designed. The children were seated securely in a baby chair. If they kicked either foot through 60 degrees this broke a lightbeam, causing a 1-second rotation of a brightly-coloured mobile. Usually, when this sort of contingency is noticed, kicking rate rises, often accompanied by smiling or excited vocalizations. The criterion adopted for having detected the relationship between kicking and the mobile turning was a 1.5 increase in each infant's personal baseline kicking rate.

These studies were basically about control and the exercise of control. There were two experimental variations:

- in *contingent* sessions, the mobile would turn if, and only if, the child kicked through the beam; in some sessions, the mobile would turn every time the child kicked, i.e., 100% of the time; in others, kicking would only work 80% of the time (with 1 in 5 kicks being 'cancelled' randomly by the computer) – real life is not always so generous as to provide a reward for effort on every occasion.

- in mixed *contingent/non-contingent* sessions, the mobile would also occasionally randomly turn by itself, around 10% of the time, even though the child had not kicked: again, this mimics real life – sometimes things happens because someone else did something, not you.

The children with DS did less well on these tasks than ND children of the same CA, as would be expected, but although generally slower to detect the relationship between their kicking and the mobile's turns, they were eventually able to solve this problem in all its various versions. In developmental terms, however, of more interest was how they responded to the *non-contingent*, 'free' turns of the mobile. Figure 6.1 (below) shows data from a baby first tested at 6 months and then at regular 3-monthly intervals until she was 2 years old. The three graphs give data from three testing sessions: at 6, 12, and 15 months.

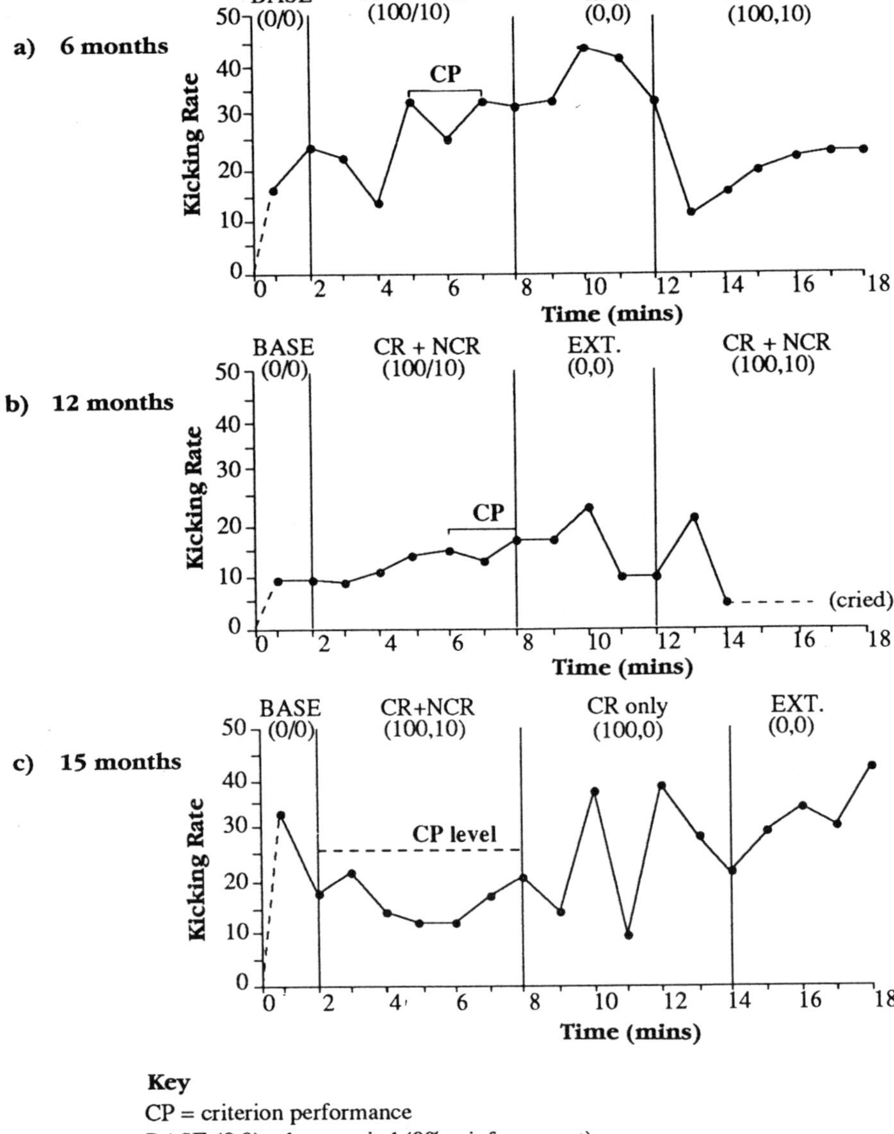


**Key**

CP = criterion performance

BASE (0,0) = base period (0% reinforcement)

CR + NCR (100,10) = 100% contingent, 10% non-contingent reinforcement

CR only (100,0) = 100% contingent, 0% non-contingent reinforcement

EXT. (0,0) = extinction period (0% reinforcement)

*Figure 6.1* Kicking activity at 6, 12 and 15 months under contingent and non-contingent schedules.

Testing sessions lasted 18 minutes. Criterion performance (CP) under a mixed schedule was achieved in the first session, at 6 months, as is clearly indicated in the sharp rise in kicking rate and again, at 12 months(paradoxically taking slightly longer at this older age – 4 rather than 3 minutes). By 15 months however, this subject simply sat watching the mobile's random turns, only occasionally bothering to kick for herself. It might seem tempting to suggest that she had just lost interest, having been exposed to the task so often. The flurries of activity when the 'free' turns were switched off (100/0) and when the mobile was turned off completely (0/0) suggest the opposite. They also confirm that she was still aware of her potential to control the mobile and was still keen to see it go round. In the non-contingent part of the session, however, she effectively relinquished her control over what was going on around her. Clearly, providing encouragement lead to a *decline* in self-generated activity at older ages; the exact opposite of what we would seek to achieve.

Table 6.1 (below) shows data from a cross-sectional study and thus from children with no prior exposure to this task. It illustrates just how differently children with DS and without DS react in this type of situation at different ages and at different stages in their development. The 16 children with DS (four each at 6, 12, 18 and 24 months) were each matched with two control ND children, one of the same CA, the other a younger ND child of the same mental age as the DS subject. There were two experimental sessions, one with, one without 'free' turns (with order of presentation counterbalanced). Although five of the older children with DS were already walking, the majority happily sat through most of both 18-minute testing sessions with very little complaint, alert and interested, and often showing considerable signs of pleasure at each rotation of the mobile. The ND children were far less tolerant and far less passive. By a developmental age of 6 months, once the contingency between their actions and the turns of the mobile had been fully

Table 6.1 Operant learning studies: mean length of cooperation (minutes) at four ages—cross-sectional data—(after Wishart 1991)

| DS age level | Session | DS Ss | CA matched Ss | MA matched Ss |
|---|---|---|---|---|
| 6 months | 1 | 14.13 | 11.00 | 10.00 |
| | 2 | 15.75 | 11.75 | 7.25 |
| 12 months | 1 | 14.50 | 3.25 | 10.25 |
| | 2 | 14.38 | 1.25 | 7.13 |
| 18 months | 1 | 15.88 | 1.00 | 2.63 |
| | 2 | 14.20 | 0.25 | 1.13 |
| 24 months | 1 | 13.50 | 0.00 | 1.13 |
| | 2 | 12.50 | 0.00 | 0.88 |

explored, they retained little interest in either task and unambiguously expressed this. Protests typically subsided immediately they were allowed out of the chair and they were still willing to cooperate in other problem-solving tasks, such as object concept tasks.

## 6.7 Object Concept Development

The second set of illustrative data is drawn from these studies of object concept development (Wishart 1988, 1993a, b). It is not necessary to go into any great detail about object concept development itself but it is important to note that the cognitive skills crucial to succeeding on these tasks are considered by many psychologists to be key ones. 'Object concept development' is a wonderfully obscure term for something that is really very simple. We all have to learn at some early point, for example, that objects exist independently of our actions, and that they continue to exist in exactly the same form even when we cannot see them or act upon them. We also have to learn that no object can be in two places at one time and that all objects have unique identities, that two objects seen at different times may look identical but are not necessarily the same object, and so on.

A series of hiding tasks of increasing complexity are used to assess how much infants understand about objects and about the physical laws that govern their movements. The easiest tasks involve hiding a small, attractive toy fully or partially under some sort of occluder, typically a cup or small cloth; in the most difficult tasks, the child must choose from two or more identical occluders, after a hiding sequence in which either the position of the toy or of the occluders has been changed.

Thirty infants with DS aged between birth and 2 years 9 months took part in a longitudinal study. We used four levels of task. Although there was already evidence to suggest that children with DS are considerably delayed in acquiring each of the stages in object concept development, we decided to try all levels of task with all ages of subject. Testing sessions were fortnightly, with the same person carrying out the testing on all occasions.

The data we shall look at here relate only to the second easiest task, a task commonly known as the *AAB* task. This task is typically solved by the average child somewhere between 8 and 10 months. A toy is hidden three times, in one of two identical occluders positioned at *A* and *B*, in the sequence *AAB*. There is no sleight of hand and the infant sees the object being hidden each time. Success requires the infant to search at *B* on the *B* trial on four out of four *AAB* trials; in longitudinal studies, success is required in two consecutive sessions. Prior to 8-10 months, the characteristic error made by ND infants is to continue to search at *A* on the *B* trial, i.e., at the place where the toy has previously been found. All children, no matter how intelligent they are, will have produced this error at some point in their development. Early experience with this sort of problem can lead to success at a younger age, but longitudinal studies have shown that the characteristic error still reliably appears in testing sessions prior to this success.

In our studies, we found that infants with DS produced exactly the same *AAB* error as ND infants but here, effectively, the similarities ended. Taking the more positive aspects of our data first, mean age of first success on this task was 7¾ months for control infants and 10½ months for infants with DS; the range of age of success is also worth noting: 7.25–14 months. The infants with DS may have taken longer to achieve their first success on this task than the ND infants but the mean age at which they did so was not far off cross-sectional norms for age of acquisition of this stage; a small number of infants in fact succeeded at surprisingly early ages. This was true of performance on higher level tasks too (see Table 6.2).

These early ages for first success were deceptive, however. Figure 6.2 shows the performance profile of one of these early achievers over a period of 12 months, between 6 and 18 months of age. It reflects the instability in development which we found to be typical of many of our young subjects with DS. This subject first succeeded on the *AAB* task at 7½ months and kept this up over five testing sessions, a period of 2 months. This could not just have been lucky guessing. Thereafter, her performance proved to be much less stable however. Her subsequent failures were sometimes the result of a refusal to engage in sufficient trials to be credited with a pass (4/4 correct searches at *B*) rather than of clearly erroneous search on any trial (*M*-). Success could sometimes be restored by hiding chocolate or a rusk instead of a toy but this strategy was not always successful (*M*+). More typically, although watching the hiding carefully

Table 6.2 Mean age of success (in months) on four levels of object concept task (after Wishart 1993a,b)

| | Task 1 | Task 2 | Task 3 | Task 4 |
|---|---|---|---|---|
| DS Children: | | | | |
| *Longitudinal data* | | | | |
| Mean age* | 7.75 | 10.50 | 19.25 | 18.0 |
| Range | 6.25-10.75 | 7.25-14.0 | 14.5-26.75 | 11.0-25.25 |
| Normally-developing Children: | | | | |
| *Longitudinal data* | | | | |
| Mean age* | 4.75 | 7.75 | 12.25 | 14.5 |
| Range | 4.0-5.75 | 4.75-8.5 | 9.25-14.25 | 10.25-17.0 |
| *Cross-sectional data* (Wishart and Bower 1984) | | | | |
| Age* at which 75% Ss passed | 5.0 | 10.0 | 15.0 | 22.0+ |

* all ages rounded up to nearest 0.25 months

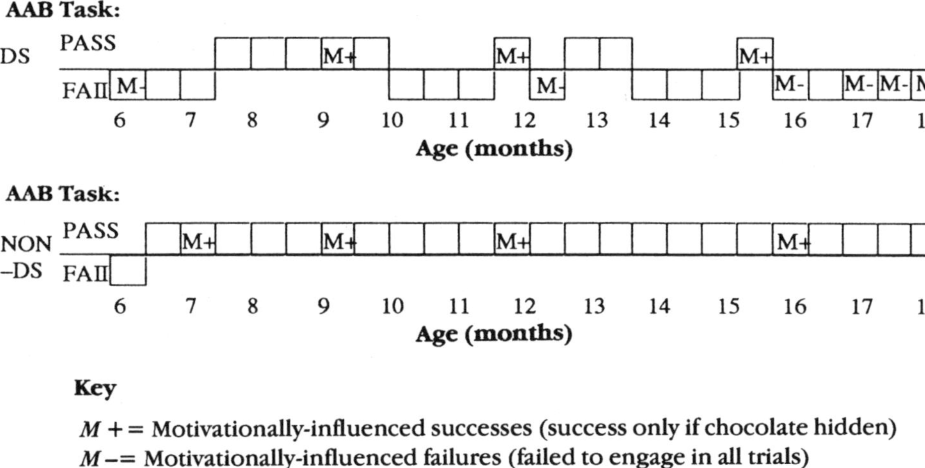


*Figure 6.2 AAB* performance profiles of two age-matched subjects.

and clearly capable of precise search, this little girl would either sweep both cups to the floor or simply pick the same cup on each trial, a very low-level strategy which at best would give a 50% return rate (and, of course would count as a 'fail').

This was not the only problem. The subjects with DS also produced counter-productive behaviours in response to tasks which were 'difficult', difficult, that is, in terms of their current developmental level. In this case, engagement was more clearly withdrawn, with difficult tasks often actively avoided after only one or two trials, either with protests or by resorting to diversionary strategies such as pretending to be very interested in something else, turning on the charm, or producing some sort of 'party-trick' (such as blowing raspberries) to divert the tester into some other, off-task activity.

These counterproductive behaviours cannot simply be written off as perfectly normal responses to being repeatedly presented with a task which is now 'easy', or being faced with a task that is just too difficult. ND children typically work hard at *all* levels of these tasks, whether they are above or below their current developmental level in terms of difficulty, with occasional lapses in interest usually easily overcome with coaxing or chocolate (see Figure 6.2). ND children usually enjoy showing off their abilities – why is it that children with DS would rather respond in a way that avoids running the risk of error, even when they should have a good chance of succeeding?

## 6.8 Behaviour in Formal Assessments

One last set of data, relating to how children with DS behave in formal assessment situations as opposed to psychological experiments, is perhaps worth looking at (Wishart and Duffy 1990; Wishart 1993a). The data already given above indicate that the differences in development in children with DS and in children without DS may be more significant than the similarities in their development. In assessing DS children, we nevertheless make great use of psychometric tests; tests that have been standardized on normally-developing children, e.g., the *Bayley Scales of Infant Development*, the *Stanford Binet Test*, or the *Wechsler Scales of Intelligence*. We then describe the child with DS in terms of his or her 'mental age' (MA), a term referring to the mental ability that would be expected in the average child of that number of years. The validity of such tests rests on the assumption that test performance will be a reasonably accurate reflection of the skills available to the child and that all children will be equally motivated to demonstrate those skills in a test setting.

Intuition alone would suggest that the child whose learning experience has been characterized by frequent failure might well approach a situation which is clearly designed to test the limits of his or her ability in a different way to a child whose experience of success and failure has been more favourable. We have found that the diversionary and delaying tactics, the non-committal responses, the misuse of social skills – the behaviours we see at younger ages – all re-appear in various guises at later ages when children are faced with standardized IQ tests. The tests we have been using are the *Mental Scale* of the *Bayley Scales of Infant Development* and the *Kaufman Assessment Battery for Children* (KABC). In some cases, when we have tested children on two separate but closely-spaced sessions, we have found performance to vary on as many as 30% of the test items presented, with children passing items previously failed and failing items previously passed. This has often meant that two very different IQs resulted from these two testing sessions, neither presumably reflecting accurately the full range of skills available to the child at that point in his or her development.

Table 6.3 shows the number of items on which performance changed between two closely-spaced sessions in a group of 18 DS children aged from 6 months to 4 years. There were 74 instances in which the children's performance improved on a test item in the second session and 91 instances in which their performance deteriorated in the second session. There is no indication of this instability in mean overall scores at any of the six age levels – these were very similar over sessions. This should sound a warning note about the confidence that can be placed in findings from studies in which subjects were 'matched' on IQ. It is not likely that all 74 instances of fail-to-pass changes can be put down to true increases in the children's competencies in the short intervening period of two weeks that separated the two testing sessions. The 91 pass-to-fail changes are less ambiguous. Clearly the required behaviour *was* already in the child's repertoire at that age but for some reason it was not reproduced in the second testing session.

Table 6.3 Test-retest stability on Bayley items at four ages (after Wishart and Duffy 1990)

| Age (months) | Testing session I | | Testing session II | | N. test items on which performance varied over two sessions | |
|---|---|---|---|---|---|---|
| | Mean raw score (AE) | | | | Fail-to-pass | Pass-to-fail |
| 6 | 55.3 | (4.5) | 53.3 | (4.5) | 12 | 19 |
| 12 | 77.3 | (7.0) | 75.6 | (7.0) | 10 | 15 |
| 18 | 100.0 | (11.0) | 99.7 | (11.0) | 11 | 13 |
| 24 | 109.0 | (13.0) | 108.7 | (13.0) | 16 | 16 |
| 36 | 131.3 | (19.0) | 130.3 | (19.0) | 12 | 15 |
| 48 | 142.3 | (22.0) | 142.3 | (22.0) | 13 | 13 |
| AE = age equivalent level (months) | | | | Totals: | 74 | 91 |

The effects on development of these fluctuations in performance profiles can be seen in Figure 6.3. Few of the Bayley items permit chance success; passes, unlike fails, are likely to be genuine. Figure 6.3 shows the relationship of MA scores to CA for a child tested twice with the Bayley every 3 months between the ages of 30 and 48 months. 'Session 1' points give the score achieved in the first of the two testing sessions presented at each age level. From these, it looks as if this child's development plateaued between 36 and 48 months, and that no developmental progress was made over this year. What will happen, though, if at each age level we credit her with all of the items on which she had scored a pass, regardless of whether this was on the first or

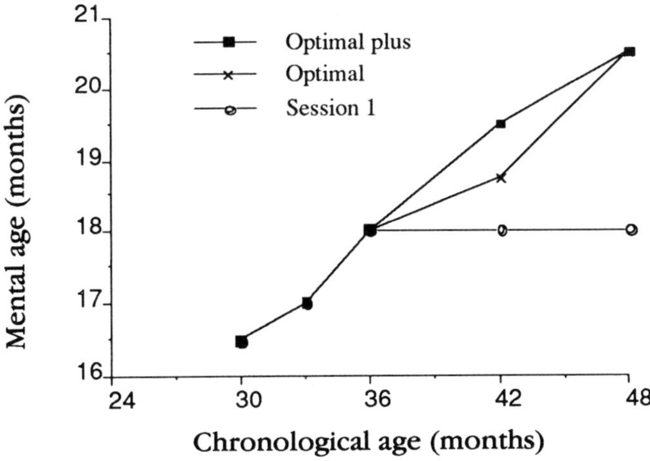


*Figure 6. 3.* The effects of instability on IQ profile.

second of the two closely-spaced sessions? From these 'optimal' scores, it is clear that new skills *were* being gained over the months but that the effects of these on her score were being cancelled out by her failure to reproduce, reliably, skills gained earlier. The 'optimal-plus' scores credit all items passed up to and including that testing session, irrespective of the reliability of those items in sessions beyond that of initial acquisition. What the 'optimal-plus' scores illustrate is the potential for constant progress – if only each new skill had been consolidated into the repertoire and used to the full. Our analyses of behaviour during testing showed that two-thirds of the pass-to-fail cases and half of the fail-to-pass cases in this group of children were associated with evidence of inadequate engagement in the task. This fits with the suggestion that psychological as well as biological factors have an important influence on how development progresses.

The degree to which these psychological factors are open to intervention remains to be determined. Although high-achieving individuals with DS may not be representative of the average. they nonetheless demonstrate that the condition does not in itself place a 'fixed' ceiling on cognitive development which is inevitably very low. Given that early intervention, professional input, and full-time schooling are now the norm, the wide differences seen in ability levels are not likely to stem simply from 'brighter' children having had more opportunities to learn than others. There *is* some evidence of a link between favourable developmental outcome and those factors which influence IQ in the rest of the population, such as level of parental education and socio-economic status, but this link is far from strong: nor is there strong evidence that variability in IQs in children with DS is closely correlated with variability in parental IQ.

Clearly psychological as well as biological factors are at work in determining developmental outcome in DS and until we gain a better understanding of how these interact we shall remain unable to explain why it is that some individuals with DS succeed in mastering so much more than others do. A closer developmental investigation of the learning process itself (rather than its products) and a more detailed analysis of the contexts in which we expect children with DS to learn could well pay rich dividends. It is also important to remember that the potential for further cognitive growth continues well beyond adolescence in those with DS (Carr 1994). It is therefore important that any lessons to be learnt from research into cognitive development in children with DS should also be appraised for their potential relevance to older age groups. Many of the psychological obstacles to learning which appear to dog early childhood must also operate in later life. At later ages, it may be even *more* likely that motivational deficits and underperformance will depress both the acquisition and development of new skills.

## Acknowledgements

This paper draws on a talk given to the National Down Syndrome Society of the United States in May 1994 and a chapter to appear in B Stratford and P Gunn (Eds) *New Approaches to Down's Syndrome*. London: Cassell (in press 1995). The research was funded by the Medical Research Council of Great Britain (Grant no. 9311518N ) and the support and encouragement of the Scottish Down's Syndrome Association is also gratefully acknowledged. Most of all, thanks are due to the many children who helped in the reported studies and who made carrying out the research so pleasurable.

## References

Bower A and Hayes A (1994) Short-term memory deficits and Down's syndrome: a comparative study. Down's Syndrome: Research and Practice 2: 47–50.

Carr J (1985) The development of intelligence. In D Lane and B Stratford (Eds) Current Approaches to Down's Syndrome, pp.167–86. London: Cassell.

Carr J (1994) Long term outcome for people with Down's syndrome. Journal of Child Psychology and Psychiatry 35: 425–39.

Cicchetti D and Beeghly M (Eds) (1990) Children with Down Syndrome: A developmental perspective. New York: Cambridge University Press.

Cunningham C (1987) Down's Syndrome: An introduction for parents. London: Souvenir Press.

Duffy L (1990) The relationship between competence and performance in early development in children with Down's syndrome. Unpublished doctoral dissertation, University of Edinburgh, Scotland.

Gibson D (1978) Down's Syndrome: The psychology of mongolism.Cambridge UK: Cambridge University Press.

Gibson D and Harris A (1988) Aggregated early intervention effects for Down Syndrome persons: Patterning and longevity of benefits. Journal of Mental Deficiency Research 32: 1–17.

Hayden AH and Dmitriev V (1975) The multidisciplinary preschool programme for Down's Syndrome children at the University of Washington Model preschool center. In BZ Friedlander, GM Sterritt and GE Kirk (Eds) The Exceptional Infant: Vol.3. Assessment and intervention, pp.193–221. New York: Brunel/Mazel.

Marcell MM and Armstrong V (1982) Auditory and visual sequential memory of Down syndrome and non-retarded children. American Journal of Mental Deficiency 87: 86–95.

Sloper P, Glenn SM and Cunningham CC (1986) The effect of intensity of training on sensori-motor development in infants with Down's syndrome. Journal of Mental Deficiency Research 30: 149–62.

Spitz HH (1986) Preventing and curing mental retardation by behavioral intervention: an evaluation of some claims. Intelligence 10: 197–207.

Uecker A, Mangan PA, Obrzut JE and Nadel L (1993) Down syndrome in neurobiological perspective: an emphasis on spatial cognition. Journal of Clinical Child Psychology 22: 266–76.

Varnhagen CK, Das JP and Varnhagen S (1987) Auditory and visual memory span: cognitive processing by TMR individuals with Down syndrome or other etiologies. American Journal of Mental Deficiency Research 91: 398–405.

Wishart JG (1988) Early learning in infants and young children with Down's Syndrome. In L Nadel (Ed) The psychobiology of Down Syndrome, pp.7–50. Boston: MIT Press.

Wishart JG (1990) Learning to learn: the difficulties faced by infants and young children with Down's Syndrome. In WI Fraser (Ed) Key issues in research in mental retardation, pp.249–61. London: Routledge.

Wishart JG (1991) Taking the initiative in learning: a developmental investigation of infants with Down's Syndrome. International Journal of Disability, Development and Education 38: 27–44.

Wishart JG (1993a) The development of learning difficulties in children with Down's syndrome. Journal of Intellectual Disability Research 37: 389–403.

Wishart JG (1993b) Learning the hard way: avoidance strategies in young children with Down's syndrome. Down's Syndrome: Research and Practice 1: 47–55.

Wishart JG (in press) Avoidant learning styles and cognitive development in young children with Down's syndrome. In B Stratford and P Gunn (Eds) New Approaches to Down's Syndrome. London: Cassell.

Wishart JG and Duffy L (1990) Instability of performance on cognitive tests in infants and young children with Down's Syndrome. British Journal of Educational Psychology 59: 10–22.

# Part Three: Psycholinguistics

# 7 Oral Language in Down's Syndrome

JEAN A RONDAL

## 7.1 Introduction

In this chapter, I will deal with four aspects of the problem:

1. The general characteristics of *language development in Down's syndrome (DS)*;
2. The levels of language function reached by *DS adolescents and adults*. One important question in this respect is whether there exists a critical period for language development in DS beyond which basic acquisitions are no longer possible;
3. The topic of *individual variation* will be addressed. I will discuss cases of advanced language abilities in DS. The *modularity hypothesis* as it applies to language function in DS will also be considered;
4. Lastly, I will turn to the question of *language specificity* comparing the language of DS subjects and mentally retarded (MR) subjects affected with other genetic syndromes.

## 7.2 Language Development in DS

### 7.2.1 Prelinguistic development

Prelinguistic development shows significant delays in DS babies. As a rule, they are less responsive to mothers' verbal stimulation than non-retarded (NR) infants of similar chronological age (CA). They tend to take the initiative less often in the interaction. Basic turn-taking skills central to future conversational exchanges are slow to develop. The type of prelinguistic phrasing that can be observed in NR babies beginning around 3 months of age, is slightly different in DS babies (Lynch *et al.* in press a). Prelinguistic phrasing is defined as intermittent babbling approximately 3 seconds long, characterized by the rhythm and structure that later underlie speech, e.g., phrase-ending syllables last longer than other syllables. DS babies display the same rhythmic organization in prelinguistic phrases as NR infants, but they take longer to finish a prelinguistic phrase (an average of more than 5 seconds compared to about 3 seconds in NR infants). This extended time frame may explain why mothers and their DS babies are often found to vocalize simultaneously (Jones 1977; Buckhalt *et al.* 1978; Berger and Cunningham 1981).

The obvious advice to mothers is to allow more time for their DS infant while managing to involve her or him gradually in the appropriate pre-conversational frame.

### 7.2.2 The sound of babbling

The sounds of babbling are mostly similar in *types* and *tokens* in NR and DS infants (Smith and Oller 1981). Their combinatory patterns may be more problematic in DS infants, however. Contrary to an earlier indication by Smith and Oller (1981), Lynch *et al.* (in press b) suggest that reduplicated babbling i.e., production of speech-like syllables: 'bababa', 'dadada' etc., is delayed and less stable in DS infants. The onset of reduplicated babbling is observed around 6 months at home and 9 months in laboratory studies in NR infants, versus 8 and 10 months, respectively, in DS infants. Reduplicated babbling may be a precursor to meaningful speech. In Lynch *et al.'s* data, the age of onset of reduplicated babbling, estimated from parent report, was significantly correlated with the DS infants' scores at 27 months CA on the *Early Social-Communication Scales* (Mundy *et al.* 1984). These scales have predictive validity with respect to subsequent development of verbal communication (Mundy *et al.* 1990). It is the case that DS negatively influences vocal development as early as the first year of life. The onset and stability of reduplicated babbling should be carefully investigated for they may yield interesting cues as to why communicative speech is markedly delayed in this syndrome.

### 7.2.3 Meaningful speech

Meaningful speech takes a long time to develop in DS. First conventional words are late to stabilize. Many DS children do not demonstrate consistent use of conventional words before three years of age. The delays in motor development and planning that are characteristic of DS (Rast and Harris 1985; Wishart 1988) bear significant correlation as likely factors contributing to the delay in speech. But there is more to it. Semantic development is also retarded in DS in proportion with the cognitive impairment characteristic of the condition. Some of the early contributors to cognitive development may be eye-contact and joint attention on the mother and child's part (Bruner 1975). DS infants exhibit delays (one month on average) in the onset of sustained eye-contact with the mother, and further delays (two months on average) in the setting of high levels of this behaviour (Berger and Cunningham 1983; Gunn *et al.* 1982). Delays in imitative verbal and gestural abilities (Gutman and Rondal 1979; Mahoney *et al.* 1981; Rondal 1980; Rondal *et al.* 1981; Sokolov 1992) may also contribute to the slow pace of development of meaningful speech production in DS. All these factors deserve careful consideration in prelinguistic intervention.

### 7.2.4 The first multiword productions

The first multiword productions that are not unanalysed formulae are observable around 4 years in DS children. Mean length of utterance (MLU) is widely used as a criterion variable for assessing language development. Up to a certain level of development almost any morphosyntactic acquisition will be directly reflected in the MLU count. Pooling together the results of a number of studies, it is possible to document MLU development in DS persons from early childhood into adulthood (see Rondal 1985, and Rondal and Comblain, in press, for a review). Figure 7.1 illustrates this development.

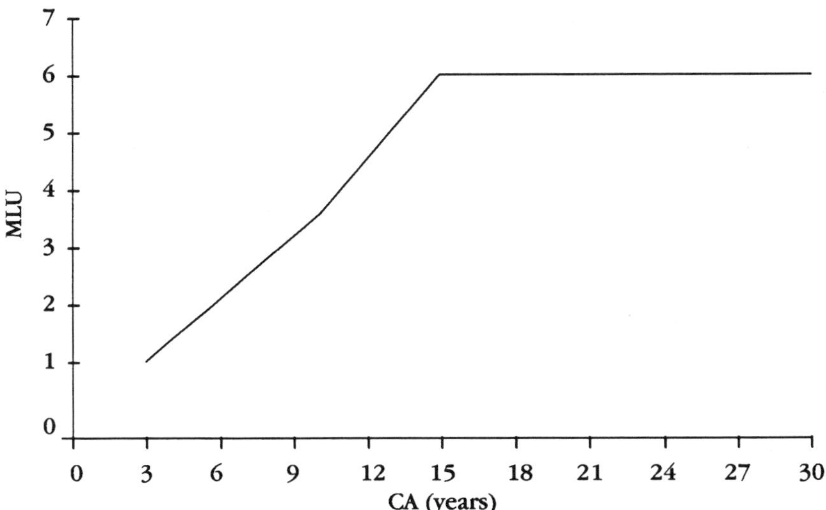


*Figure 7.1* Evolution of mean length of utterance in Down's syndrome. MLU is computed in number of words plus grammatical morphemes (according to the procedure outlined in Brown (1973) and Rondal *et al.* (1986))

As shown in Figure 7.1, MLU development in DS shows a good linear relationship with CA until early adolescence despite the existence of an important delay. I will come back later to the plateau beyond 15 years CA. In comparison with DS children, NR children reach MLU levels of 5 units and more around 6 years. In conversational speech between NR adults, MLU values are often close to 12. The slowness and limitation of MLU development in DS correspond to lasting shortcomings in morpho-syntax.

Productive use of grammatical words (articles, prepositions, pronouns, conjunctions, auxiliaries) and morphological marking of gender, number, tense, mode and aspect are limited. Most DS subjects are restricted to short monopropositional sentences with correct word order. Subordinate clauses are rare. Even at corresponding MLU levels, DS children may not demonstrate exactly the same kind of syntax as NR peers (see Rondal 1978). For example, when matched for MLU with NR children, DS children tend to use fewer complex verb groups and advanced types of indefinite pronouns. Corresponding limitations can be observed in the understanding of grammatical structures (Bartel *et al.* 1973).

### 7.2.5 Progmatics and Communication

There is a growing literature on language pragmatics and linguistic communication in MR (see Rosenberg and Abbeduto 1993 for a review). It is known that young DS children (1–4 years of age) use one-word utterances efficiently to request interesting objects located out of reach (Greenwald and Leonard 1979). Several studies report few differences between MA-matched NR and DS children in the frequency of speech acts, e.g., question–answer, assertion, suggestion, request, command (Owens and MacDonald 1982; Coggins *et al.* 1983). But important limitations exist in the use of the linguistic forms that NR people find appropriate for the expression of particular speech acts. For example, DS children have difficulty in using conventional forms for 'softening' their requests or rendering them more 'polite' by some means such as indirect requesting.

Conservational turn-taking does not constitute a problem for older DS subjects. Their turn-taking behaviour is systematic and rule-governed. Topic contribution and topic continuation in DS persons have not been studied in detail. It is likely that DS individuals, as well as other MR individuals, have keen desires to keep a topic going when conversing and to contribute significantly to conversations. But they often lack the language skills and the relevant knowledge to do so.

In a nutshell, the language of DS individuals is formally restricted but semantically and pragmatically appropriate to limited cognitive and social demands.

### 7.2.6 Is DS language simply delayed or qualitatively different?

The question was raised years ago, (Yoder and Miller 1972), whether language development in MR children is a delayed version of normal language development or whether it shows qualitatively different patterns. It is possible now to give a precise answer to this question based on the large number of studies conducted over the last 25 years (see Rondal and Edwards, in press, for a review). Clearly, language development in DS children is not just a slow-motion version of normal language development. From the early stages on, there are noticeable differences with NR children, including particular limitations and distortions for which we do not have adequate explanations yet. Also, language development in DS is never complete. It plateaus at various times depending on the particular aspect considered. A strict delay-difference framework is not appropriate for describing language development in MR individuals (Rondal 1984, 1985, 1987). But language development in DS subjects (as well as in other MR categories) is not exotic either. Most importantly, the sequence of developmental steps is the same in DS and NR children (*similar sequence hypothesis*). It is appropriate therefore to apply a developmental perspective to the study of language in DS as well as to guiding remedial work with these individuals.

## 7.3 Language Functioning in DS Adolescents and Adults

We have developed a sense of life-continuation regarding DS persons. It is imperative that systematic studies be conducted to specify the expectations one may have regarding the abilities of DS adults. Life expectancy in DS is estimated to be about 50 years. It is expected that between 1990 and 2010, the number of DS persons over 40 years old will increase by 75%, and over 50 old years by 200% (Steffelaar and Evenhuis 1989). Table 7.1 summarizes additional information on life expectancy in DS persons.

One important question is: How does the language of DS adolescents and adults compare with that of DS children? It relates to the problem of the existence of a critical period for first language acquisition as raised by Lenneberg (1967). Lenneberg's conclusion was that due to the maturational calendar of the brain, no basic language development could be possible beyond puberty. He claimed to have observations from DS

Table 7.1 Life expectancy in persons with Down's syndrome[1].

| Year | DS population | Normal population |
|---|---|---|
| 1929 | 9 years | |
| 1947 | 12-15 years | |
| 1961 | 18 years | |
| 1988 | 44% > 60 years | 86.4% > 60 years |
| | 13.8% > 68 years | 78.4% > 68 years |

[1] Irrespective of sex.

subjects supporting this hypothesis (Lenneberg *et al.* 1964). We now have more systematic data pertaining to the problem and are in a better position to assess the validity of the critical period hypothesis for first language acquisition.

In NR individuals, crucial indications are available from Genie, a modern-day 'wild child' who was kept away from social contact for most of her first 13 years (Curtiss 1977). When she was discovered, she understood only a few words and did not speak. From that time, she developed relatively rapidly in the cognitive area and enriched substantially her referential lexicon and semantics. But, the acquisition of grammatical rules and their use in complex utterances never followed. To date, Genie's expressive language has remained grammatically underdeveloped. Word order is globally appropriate but the utterances lack bound and free grammatical morphemes. Advanced syntactic devices are missing. Other cases exhibiting the same general pattern have been documented. For example, consider Chelsea, a hearing-impaired adult of normal intelligence who first attempted to acquire spoken language in her 30s, following successful auditory amplification (Curtiss 1988). Chelsea's lexical knowledge progressed regularly (she scored above the 12th-grade level on the Productive Word Association Subtest of the *Clinical Evaluation of Language Functions* (Semmel and Wiig 1980). In contrast, her ability to combine words into utterances remained extremely limited resulting in multiword combinations being ungrammatical most of the time.

Further data suggest a critical period for the development of grammar setting mechanisms. Mayberry *et al* (1983) showed that individuals who acquired American Sign Language (ASL) as adolescents perform worse on tasks assessing grammatical knowledge in ASL than individuals who acquired this language in childhood. Corresponding indications were published by Newport (1990, 1992).

The data argue in favour of the existence of neuropsychological mechanisms devoted to the grammatical and phonological (i.e., the computational) aspects of language (Chomsky 1981). Such mechanisms are tied to the left-cerebral hemisphere and develop according to strong maturational constraints. There is no indication that the development of semantic, lexical and pragmatic skills (i.e., the more conceptual and social aspects of language) are characterized by similar temporal constraints.

The critical period for computational language development is likely to have modular characteristics: expressed differently, there may be an aggregate of particular phenomena coinciding partially in time. The critical phonological period may terminate around 7 years of age. Judging from available data on the difference in vocal capacity between congenitally deaf individuals or individuals having become deaf early in life (i.e., before about 2 years of age (Menyuk 1977)), and subjects with deafness that occurred later in life, there is probably an earlier critical period for voice setting and control. The ending of the critical period for morpho-syntax may be around 14 years. Hurford (1991) suggests that the main determinant for the end point(s) of the critical period(s) is 'the consequences of the interplay of genetic factors influencing life-history characteristics in relation to language acquisition'.

Assuming that the evolutionary constraints advocated by Hurford (1991) apply equally to MR individuals (including DS individuals), it can be predicted that no basic computational language development will be possible beyond 14–15 years in these subjects. Training effects may still be induced later because critical periods do not end abruptly. But the effect of training will be at a markedly increased cost with advancing chronological age. Development in the conceptual aspects of language may continue during adolescence and beyond, in proportion to a possible continued growth in mental age (MA) (Fisher and Zeaman 1970; Berry *et al.* 1984).

As I have documented elsewhere (see Rondal and Comblain, in press), the above predictions are supported by facts. Observing language evolution in MR from late childhood on to adulthood, little structural progress is obvious in the phonological and morphosyntactic aspects of language beyond late childhood. One of the few changes that I was able to document concerns a limited improvement in sentence understanding (for example, coordinate, negative and relative clauses). It is not clear, however, whether this improvement reflects a genuine albeit limited linguistic progress or rather a better ability to deal with experimental tasks.

In contrast to phonology and morpho-syntax, continued improvement beyond childhood seems to be generally the case for referential lexical abilities and pragmatics.

The implications of the above findings for language intervention are straightforward. Phonological and morpho-syntactic training should be programmed at maximal rate during childhood. Adequate potential for further development may no longer be there beyond 14 years in these areas (possibly earlier for phonological development). Semantic, lexical and pragmatic training should also be performed intensely during childhood, but they can be continued profitably in adolescence and early adulthood. For those language aspects, there is still adequate potential for development beyond childhood.

## 7.4 Individual Variation in DS Language

Language development and functioning in DS has been noted for presenting important inter-individual variations. This variability has only begun to be studied systematically. In one of the few studies available, Fishler and Koch (1991) report anecdotal observations regarding 'unusually good quality of speech' (p.93) in mosaic DS children, contrasting with the speech of children with regular trisomy 21. In contrast to the conclusion of the authors, however, there is no objective basis in the study for claiming that mosaic DS subjects have 'relatively normal speech' (p.345). Mosaic DS subjects could have higher referential lexical and semantic levels in proportion with their more advanced cognitive capacities but this has still to be proven (Gibson 1978).

Other studies have documented rare cases of extreme variation in the language capacity of non-mosaic DS individuals. Seagoe (1965) reported the case of Paul, a DS man whom she followed from 11 to 43 years. Paul had an excellent command of written language expression and reading. Average number of words per written sentence varied from 7 to 12 words. Sentence construction was grammatical. Unfortunately, Seagoe did not report on Paul's oral language.

More recently, I have documented the case of a French-speaking DS woman with regular trisomy 21, named Françoise (Rondal 1994a, b, 1995). She has a non-verbal IQ of 60 (Wechsler Adult Intelligence Scale). Non-verbal MA is 5 years 8 months (Epreuves Différentielles d'Efficience Intellectuelle, Perron-Borelli and Misès 1974). She was classified late preoperational on the Piagetian levels of intellectual development. Françoise thus presents a cognitive development only moderately superior to the one typically reached by regular DS subjects. In contrast Françoise's oral language is most unusual. Her articulation and phoneme discrimination are correct in all respects. Lexical development is only moderately retarded. Expressive and receptive morpho-syntax are well advanced, being virtually normal by NR adult standards. Her conversational MLU is 12.24. She produces grammatical sentences counting up to 50 words. Problems can be identified at the level of discourse organization, however. Her longer texts often lack cohesion, but on the whole the language is pragmatically adequate.

Particularly astonishing is Françoise's capacity to deal with complex morpho-syntactic structures. On several psycholinguistic tasks specially devised to test advanced morpho-syntactic competence, she proved able to process correctly complex linguistic structures such as:

1. Reversible relative clauses introduced by pronouns *qui* or *que,* whether embedded or derived on the right of the main clause;
2. Causal subordinate clauses introduced by the conjunctive locution *parce que,* whether the subordinate clause precedes or follows the main clause;
3. Temporal subordinate clauses, whether the clause order matches the order of events in reality or not;
4. The mechanism of coreference in the case of anaphoric personal pronouns, even when the distance between pronoun and nominal coreferent amounts to seven words;

5. Declarative passive sentences varying in plausibility and plausible reversibility, including sentences low in semantic transitivity, the correct comprehension of which is late to stabilize in NR subjects (Hopper and Thompson 1980).

Most remarkably, Françoise could correctly identify the underlying grammatical subject or the underlying grammatical object in unrealistic sentences (e.g., *Le livre est imaginé par la boît* – The book is imagined by the box), that is, without lexical-pragmatical help; and even in unrealistic sentences that would turn realistic were they reversed (e.g., *Le monsieur est imaginé par le livre* – The man is imagined by the book), that is, going against 'natural' pragmatic interpretive tendency to reverse the sentence. Language-regular DS subjects do not even approach Françoise's demonstrated level of grammatical functioning.

Vallar and Papagno (1993) have published the case of another young DS woman showing exceptional linguistic talents. FF, as she is named in the report, is a 23-year-old Italian woman with trisonomy 21 who demonstrates good acquisition of the Italian language. She was also able to learn some English and French. Unfortunately, Vallar and Papagno's report is not precise enough to evaluate properly the extent of FF's grammatical talent.

It is not known whether there are other DS individuals with exceptional language abilities. We ought to inquire more into this matter and specify better the range of individual variation in DS.

Corresponding cases of exceptional language in non-DS MR subjects have been reported. They concern half-a-dozen subjects (Williams syndrome (WS), hydrocephaly, and MR of unknown etiology). I have summarized these cases elsewhere (Rondal 1994b, 1995). They all present the same global pattern, i.e., normal-like phonology and advanced morpho-syntactic abilities in the face of limited cognitive means. Lexical capacity is consistent with cognitive level, except in the WS cases where it is superior. Pragmatic regulations and social-communicative uses of language often make problems to these subjects. Some of them have poorly developed topic-maintenance skills, are only moderately sensitive to the interests of the interlocutors, and do not seem to be very concerned with the need to be relevant.

We need to explain the fact that advanced and even normal-like phonological and grammatical development is possible in spite of severe cognitive deficits. This most difficult question calls for an extended discussion that cannot be reproduced here (see Rondal 1994b). In the case of Françoise, my DS subject with 'normal' phonological and morpho-syntactic functioning, language training, cognitive development and short-term memory could be ruled out as major explanatory variables. The same negative interpretation is also in order for the other exceptional language cases documented in the literature; except perhaps in the case of FF for whom Vallar and Papagno (1993) claim a particular causal role of working memory which is largely unsubstantiated in my opinion. Regarding DS cases such as Françoise, the following explanatory suggestion can be made. We know that the genes in genetic syndromes such as DS are normal (Epstein 1991). If Chomsky and others are right in postulating the existence of genetically coded grammatical information in humans, and Liberman and others are right regarding genetically coded phonetic information, the same innate language basis must be recognized in all MR subjects with genetic or non-genetic syndromes (Liberman and Mattingly 1985, 1989). If one refuses the existence of an innate substantial language basis in humans, one has at least to admit that brain structures specialized for language have an innate determinism and that this determinism also applies to MR individuals. In language-regular MR subjects, therefore, either the genetically coded language information is not expressed phenotypically, or the devoted brain structures do not develop so as to permit advanced language functioning – or both may occur. Language-exceptional MR subjects escape this dramatic situation for reasons that we do not know but should be actively trying to discover.

In summary, I tend to locate the explanation of the exceptional cases of language development in MR individuals at the convergence locus of genetic information and epigenetic structural development. Comparing regular and exceptional cases in MR individuals at the neurological level should supply us with important information on genotype-phenotype relations from the language point of view.

As I have argued elsewhere (Rondal 1994b), the language-exceptional cases are also most important from another theoretical point of view, i.e., with respect to the time-honoured question of the relation between non-verbal cognition and language.

The dissociations documented above falsify the Piagetian position as well as other 'cognition-drives-grammar' positions – this was the competition model proposed by MacWhinney (MacWhinney 1987; Bates and MacWhinney 1987); and Langacker's (1987) so-called cognitive grammar, etc. These positions maintain that grammatical development deductively follows from cognitive regulations. The language-exceptional MR subjects have the same cognitive limitations as language-regular MR subjects, but they develop extensively with respect to the computational aspects of language. The conclusion is that cognitive models cannot account for the exceptional cases of computational language development in MR. By extension, it can be proposed that these models offer no solid explanation of the same aspects of language development in NR children.

The exceptional cases studied reveal important dissociations between language components: phonology and morpho-syntax, on the one hand; lexicon, semantics and pragmatics, on the other. These dissociations correspond to Chomsky's (1981) distinction between computational and conceptual (and social) aspects of language. In these cases, the preserved computational components of language are fairly independent from the severely limited non-verbal cognitive capacities exhibited by the subjects. In contrast, the conceptual components of language more directly reflect the MR subjects' cognitive limitations.

I have reviewed (Rondal 1994b) a large number of data on the modularity status of language coming from other works in patholinguistics, e.g., studies with specifically language impaired children, neuropsychological studies of regular aphasias and primary degenerative diseases, progressive aphasias, Pick's disease, Alzheimer's disease. Work in theoretical linguistics (Chomsky 1984), psycholinguistics and neurolinguistics in the last decade has led to a reconceptualization of the very notion of language. A global concept of language appears too encompassing. It may be that language normality has the general effect (or is largely the effect) of 'holding the various language components together' with the consequence that they appear more united than they are. In other words, language components interact with each other in normal functioning, but they are not intrinsically united as the dissociations uncovered by pathological processes demonstrate.

Exactly what type of modular organization is involved in language is not clear at the present time. Moscovitch and Umilta (1990) propose to define language as a type-II modular organization, i.e., a system consisting of a collection of modules whose structure is innately specified and whose output is synthesized by a devoted non-modular processor, i.e., a processor only able to deal with particular modules. Type-II modules are capable of modification through learning, not just by maturation. They may integrate type-I or Fodorian modules i.e., the largely encapsulated mechanisms of speech perception, word recognition and syntactic parsing, in addition to other modular subsystems (Fodor 1983). Ongoing research, particularly in language pathologies and cognitive neuropsychology, will allow us to develop the modular theory further.

The modular conception of language has important implications for remediation with language-impaired children. If the basic organization of language entails considerable autonomy between components, and if the computational aspects of language are largely independent from general cognition, then little should be expected from global remediation strategies. Many remedial programmes in existence are based on the assumption that training cognitive prerequisites to morpho-syntax gives the best chance of improving the language of MR children. Judging from the preceding discussion, such an assumption may be inappropriate and the remedial activities based on this premise doomed to failure. This may explain, at least partially, the limited success of grammar-teaching programmes over the years (Snyder-McLean and

McLean 1987). I am not claiming that it is unproductive to base all language remediation on cognition. The strategy is correct with respect to the conceptual aspects of language. And language remediation in these areas has generally been successful. I suggest that for phonology and morpho-syntax, the remediative efforts should concentrate more on training the computational structures themselves. Professionals ought to stop expecting that supplying a relevant cognitive basis will be sufficient to build and stabilize formal linguistic structures. Also, remediation should be conceived more in conformity with the constraints of the critical periods for linguistic acquisitions. Lastly, as I will now explain, the language remediative efforts should take more into account the language specificity of MR syndromes.

## 7.5 Language Syndromic Specificity in Mental Retardation

People are used to thinking that language development and functioning is mostly similar across MR syndromes at corresponding psychometric levels. However, recent studies force us to reconsider this belief. Space is not available to deal fully with this intricate question. The interested reader should see Rondal (in press) and particularly Rondal and Edwards (in press). Relevant data are still insufficient in quantity; but for a small number of syndromes, it is already possible to reach conclusions.

The latest classification manual from the American Association on Mental Retardation (AAMR) lists more than 400 entities and syndromes causing mental retardation (Luckasson *et al.* 1992). The genetic syndromes alone number 43. Presently, only a few of these syndromes have been studied from a speech and language point of view. Down's syndrome, of course, is well known, but there is no good reason to assume that it is the prototypical entity for moderate and severe MR. Actually, it has been claimed repeatedly that DS as a condition is more detrimental to language than other etiological entities of MR (Zisk and Bialer 1967; Fowler 1990; Kernan 1990). There could be meaningful differences in language capacities between DS and other MR entities. This is indeed what the beginning of specialized literature on the question reveals.

A number of language studies have been conducted in recent years on Williams syndrome (WS), a rare congenital metabolic disorder (1 case in 10 000 or 20 000 live births) that is associated with hemizygous deletion including the elastin locus at chromosome 7q11.23. Many, perhaps most WS subjects (the exact range of variation in the syndrome has not been documented yet), have excellent referential lexical and good productive morpho-syntactic abilities in spite of limited cognitive means (IQ varies from 40 to 60; Arnold *et al.* 1985). Some WS subjects seem to enjoy exceptional lexical abilities, cursorily using and comprehending low-

Table 7.2 Three MR syndromic profiles for speech and language

| Language aspect | Down | Syndromes<br>Williams | Fragile-X<br>(affected males) |
|---|---|---|---|
| Phonetico-phonological | -- | + | -- |
| Lexical | - | ++ | + |
| Thematic semantic | + | + | ? |
| Morpho-syntactic | -- | (comprehension?) | - |
| Pragmatic | + | -- | - |
| Discursive | -- | + | - |

*Key* +(+): relative strength; -(-): relative weakness; ?: insufficient data

frequency vocabulary items e.g., brontosaurus, sea lion, sabertoothed-tiger (Bellugi *et al.* 1988). Pragmatics is their area of major weakness. They often have difficulties with topic introduction, topic maintenance, turn taking, and maintaining appropriate eye contact. WS subjects sometimes appear to be talking nonsense and will mimic others. Their speech may be socially inappropriate and repetitive with incessant irrelevant questions. It is not clear whether their language comprehension at the morpho-syntactic level matches their productive capacity. WS subjects may echo or repeat phrases and sentences spoken by the interlocutor, apparently with limited understanding of what the person said. Articulation and speech fluency are good although occasional hoarse voice and hypernasality can be observed.

The syndrome termed 'Fragile-X' (F-XS), an X-linked disorder, has also motivated a number of research studies in recent years (Mulley *et al.* 1992). Although the situation of the affected and the carrier females is less clear (see Dykens *et al.* 1994) the language picture for the affected males may be summarized as follows:

1. Speech is often repetitive, with cluttering and fluctuating rates.
2. Unusual voice effects, dysrythmia, echolalia, speech impulsiveness and poor intelligibility have been noted (Newell *et al.* 1983; Borghraef *et al.* 1987).
3. F-XS males also frequently omit or substitute vocalic or consonant phonemes (Vilkman *et al.* 1988). Less is known about their morpho-syntactic skills. Syntaxis is an area of possible deficit in these subjects (Sudhalter *et al.* 1991).
4. The language of F-XS males also seems to be pragmatically limited. They may exhibit deviant repetitive language either at the level of the phrase, the sentence, or the topic, e.g., talking incessantly about one single topic.

A number of other genetic or metabolic syndromes leading to MR are currently the object of much research interest from a medical, physiological, or cytogenetic point of view. They are, for example, Prader-Willi syndrome, phenylketonuria, the prenatal effects of maternal hyperphenylalaninemia, and Cri-du-chat syndrome. To date, however, these syndromes have been little studied from a language point of view.

Table 7.2 briefly summarizes language data for the three genetic syndromes most studied with regard to language development – DS, WS and affected F-XS males.

The initial systematization offered in Table 7.2 is sufficient to realize that the language profiles of DS, WS and F-XS individuals differ substantially in ways not previously stated. The syndromic differences have little to do with the psychometric levels of retardation in each syndrome.

It is probably too early to propose explanations for language syndrome specificity. But some reasonable speculation is permitted. In my opinion, the syndromic variation corresponds in the first place to syndrome differences in neurodevelopment and brain structures. DS subjects are known to have central nervous system dysfunction secondary to abnormal brain development at the pre-, peri-, and postnatal stages of brain maturation. The examination of DS brains shows a reduction in weight of the brain hemispheres, brain stem, and cerebellum, delay in myelinisation, primarily in the development of the association cortex, reduction in the number of neurons in the whole cerebral cortex but more particularly in some cortical layers (Ross *et al.* 1984; Wisniewski 1990; Wisniewski *et al.* 1986). It may be suspected that in DS the arrest of neuronal proliferation and differentiation takes place around birth (Nadel 1986). It is also likely that the DS persons' reduced synaptic density and abnormal synaptic morphology (e.g., reduced contacts and lower surface areas of synaptic contacts) originate in pre- and postnatal stages of neuronal development (Wisniewski and Kida 1994). This is most unfortunate judging from neurodevelopmental data showing major postnatal growth of the 'neuropil' in normal subjects (growth of neurons and densification of the matrix of axons, dendrites, and synapses that lie between the nerve cell bodies in the brain) (Purves 1988, 1995). The abnormal neurogenesis in DS most likely reflects genetically determined altered brain programming.

The multidisciplinary study of intersyndromic differences at the neurological level promises significant advances in the explanation of basic language mechanisms and disorders. Such studies have started. For example, Bellugi and her team, at the Salk Institute, are actively pursuing a line of psycholinguistic, neuropsychological, neuroanatomical and neurophysiological analyses. Their early results cannot be discussed here for lack of space (see Bellugi *et al.* 1990; Wang *et al.* 1992; Galaburda *et al.* 1994; Wang 1992). These studies suggest the existence of important neurological differences between syndromes that may explain the particular fractionation of language functions observed.

The comparative language studies analysed indicate that the label 'specific' can be attached to systemic aspects of the language of MR subjects with particular syndromes. This is important for research, as said, but also for education. The syndrome specificity claim implies that only intervention strategies tailored to the particular patterns of relative strengths and weaknesses of people with various MR syndromes, will have the best chances to be maximally efficient. It is in that direction that remediation programmes should be heading.

## Reference

Arnold R, Yule W and Martin N (1985) The psychological characteristics of infantile hypercalcaemia: A preliminary investigation. Developmental Medicine and Child Neurology 27: 49–59.

Bartel N, Bryen S and Keehn S (1973) Language comprehension in the moderately retarded child. Exceptional Children 39: 375–82.

Bates E and MacWhinney B (1987) Competition, variation, and language learning. In B MacWhinney (Ed) Mechanisms of language acquisition, pp.157–93. Hillsdale NJ: Erlbaum.

Bellugi U, Bihrle A, Jernigan T, Trauner D and Doherty S (1990) Neuropsychological, neurological and neuroanatomical profile of Williams syndrome. American Journal of Medical Genetics Supplement 6: 115–25.

Bellugi U, Marks S, Bihrle A and Sabo H (1988) Dissociation between language and cognitive functions in Williams syndrome. In D Bishop and K Mogford (Eds) Language development in exceptional circumstances, pp.177–89. London: Churchill Livingstone.

Berger J and Cunningham CC (1981) The development of eye contact between mothers, normal and Down's syndrome infants. Developmental Psychology 17: 678–89.

Berger J and Cunningham CC (1983) The development of early vocal behaviours and interactions in Down syndrome and non-handicapped infant-mother. Developmental Psychology 19: 322–31.

Berry P, Groenweg G, Gibson D and Brown R (1984) Mental development of adults with Down syndrome. American Journal of Mental Deficiency 89: 252–6.

Borghgraef M, Fryns JP, Dielkens A, Pyck K and Van den Berghe H (1987) Fragile X syndrome: A study of the psychological profile in 23 prepubertal patients. Clinical Genetics 32: 179–86.

Bruner JS (1975) From communication to language – A psychological perspective. Cognition 3: 256–87.

Buckhalt J, Rutherford R and Goldberg I (1978) Verbal and non-verbal interaction of mothers with their Down's syndrome and non-retarded infants. American Journal of Mental Deficiency 82: 337–43.

Chomsky N (1981) Lectures on government and binding. Dordrecht Netherlands: Foris.

Chomsky N (1984) Modular approaches to the study of mind. San Diego CA: San Diego State University Press.

Coggins T, Carpenter R and Owings N (1983) Examining early intentional communication in Down's syndrome and nonretarded children. British Journal of Disorders of Communication 18: 99–107.

Curtiss S (1977) Genie: A psycholinguistic study of a modern-day 'wild child'. New York: Academic Press.

Curtiss S (1988) The special talent of grammar acquisition. In L Obler and D Fein (Eds) The exceptional brain, pp.364–86. New York: Guilford.

Dykens E, Hodapp R and Leckman J (1994) Behavior and development in Fragile X syndrome. London: Sage Publications.

Epstein C (1991) Aneuploidy and morphogenesis. in C Epstein (Ed) The morphogenesis of Down syndrome, pp.1–18. New-York: Wiley-Liss.

Fisher M and Zeaman D (1970) Growth and decline in retardate intelligence. In N Ellis (Ed) International review of research in mental retardation 4: 151–91. New York: Academic Press.

Fishler K and Koch R (1991) Mental development in Down syndrome mosaicism. American Journal on Mental Retardation 96: 345–51.

Fodor J (1983) The modularity of mind. Cambridge MA: MIT Press.

Fowler A (1990) Language abilities in children with Down syndrome: Evidence for a specific syntactic delay. In D Cicchetti and M Beeghly (Eds) Children with Down syndrome. A developmental perspective, pp.302–28. New York: Cambridge University Press.

Galaburda A, Wang P, Bellugi U and Rossen M (1994) Cytoarchitectonic anomalies in a genetically based disorder: Williams syndrome. Cognitive Neuroscience and Neuropsychology 5: 753–7.

Gibson D (1978) Down's syndrome. The psychology of mongolism. New York: Cambridge University Press.

Greenwald C and Leonard L (1979) Communicative and sensorimotor development of Down's syndrome children. American Journal of Mental Deficiency 84: 296–303.

Gunn P, Berry P and Andrews R (1982) Looking behavior of Down's syndrome infants. American Journal of Mental Deficiency 87: 344–7.

Gutman A and Rondal JA (1979) Verbal operants in mother's speech to nonretarded and Down's syndrome children matched for linguistic level. American Journal of Mental Deficiency 83: 446–52.

Hopper P and Thompson S (1980) Transitivity in grammar and discourse. Language 56: 251–99.

Hurford J (1991) The evolution of the critical period for language acquisition. Cognition 40: 159–201.

Jones O (1977) Mother-child communication with pre-linguistic Down's syndrome and normal infants. In H Schaffer (Ed) Studies in mother-infant interaction, pp.126–49. New York: Academic.

Kernan K (1990) Comprehension of syntactically indicated sequence by Down's syndrome and other mentally retarded adults. Journal of Mental Deficiency Research 34: 169–78.

Langacker R (1987) Foundations of cognitive grammar. Stanford CA: Stanford University Press.

Lenneberg E (1967) Biological foundations of language. New York: Wiley.

Lenneberg E, Nichols I and Rosenberg E (1964) Primitive stages of language development in mongolism. In D McRioch and E Weinstein (Eds) Disorders of communication. Proceedings of the Association for research in Nervous and Mental Disease 17: 119–37. Baltimore: Williams and Wilkins.

Liberman A and Mattingly I (1985) The motor theory of speech perception revised. Cognition 21: 1–36.
Liberman A and Mattingly I (1989) A specialization for speech perception. Science 243: 489–94.
Lynch M, Oller D, Steffens M and Buder E (in press a) Phrasing in prelinguistic vocalizations. Developmental Psychology.
Lynch M, Oller D, Steffens M, Levine S, Basinger D and Umbel V (in press b) The onset of speech-like vocalizations in infants with Down syndrome. American Journal of Mental Retardation.
Luckasson R, Coulter D, Polloway E, Reiss S, Shalock K, Snell M, Spitalnik D and Stark J (1992) Mental retardation, definition, classification, and systems of supports. Washington DC: American Association on Mental Retardation.
MacWhinney B (1987) The competition model. In B MacWhinney (Ed) Mechanisms of language acquisition, pp.249-308. Hilldsdale NJ: Erlbaum.
Mahoney G, Glover A and Finger I (1981) Relationship between language and sensorimotor development of Down syndrome and nonretarded children. American Journal of Mental Deficiency 86: 21–7.
Mayberry R, Fisher S, Hatfield N (1983) Sentence repetition in American Sign Language. In J Kyle and B Woll (Eds) Language in sign: International perspective on sign language, pp.206–14. London: Croom Helm.
Menyuk P (1977) Language and maturation. Cambridge MA: MIT Press.
Moscovitch M and Umilta C (1990) Modularity and neuropsychology: Modules and central processes in attention and memory. In M Schwartz (Ed) Modular deficits in Alzheimer-type dementia, pp.1–59. Cambridge MA: MIT Press.
Mulley J, Kerr B, Stevenson R and Lubs H (1992) Nomenclature guidelines for X-linked mental retardation. American Journal of Medical Genetics 43: 383–91.
Mundy P, Seibert J and Hogan A (1984) Relationship between sensorimotor and early communication abilities in developmentally delayed children. Merrill-Palmer Quarterly 30: 33–48.
Mundy P, Sigman M and Kasari C (1990) A longitudinal study of joint attention and language development in autistic children. Journal of Autism and Developmental Disorders 20: 115–28.
Nadel L (1986) Down syndrome in neurobiological perspective. In C Epstein (Ed) The neurobiology of Down syndrome, pp.239–51. New York: Raven Press.
Newell K, Sanborn B and Hagerman R (1983) Speech and language dysfunction in the fragile X syndrome. In R Hagerman and P McBogg (Eds) The fragile X syndrome: Diagnosis, biochemistry, and intervention, pp.175–220. Dillon CO: Spectra.
Newport E (1990) Maturational constraints on language learning. Cognitive Science 14: 11–28.
Newport E (1992) Contrasting conception of the critical period for language. In S Carey and R Gelman (Eds) The epigenesis of mind: Essays on biology and cognition, pp.111–30. Hillsdale NJ: Erlbaum.
Owens R and MacDonald J (1982) Communicative uses of the early speech of nondelayed and Down syndrome children. American Journal of Mental Deficiency 86: 503–10.
Perron-Borelli M and Misès, R (1974) Epreuves Différentielles d'Efficience Intellectuelle. Issy-les-Moulineaux, France: Editions Scientifiques et Psychologiques.
Purves D (1988) Body and brain: A trophic theory of neural connections. Cambridge MA: Harvard University Press.
Purves D (1995) Neural activity and the growth of the brain. Cambridge UK: Cambridge University Press.

Rast M and Harris S (1985) Motor control in infants with Down syndrome. Developmental Medicine and Child Neurology 27: 675–85.

Rondal JA (1978) Developmental sentence scoring procedure and the delay-difference question in language development of Down's syndrome children. Mental Retardation 16: 169–71.

Rondal JA (1980) Verbal imitation by Down syndrome and nonretarded children. American Journal of Mental Deficiency 85: 318–21.

Rondal JA (1984) Linguistic and prelinguistic development in moderate and severe mental retardation. In J Dobbing, A Clarke, J Corbett, J Hogg and R Robinson (Eds) Scientific studies in mental retardation, pp.323–45. London: The Royal Society of Medicine and MacMillan.

Rondal JA (1985) Adult-child interaction and the process of language acquisition. New York: Praeger.

Rondal JA (1987) Language development and mental retardation. In W Yule and M Rutter (Eds) Language development and disorders, pp.248–61. Oxford: Blackwell.

Rondal JA (1994a) Exceptional cases of language development in mental retardation: The relative autonomy of language as a cognitive system. In H Tager-Flusberg (Ed) Constraints on language acquisition: Studies of atypical children, pp.155–74. Hillsdale NJ: L. Erlbaum.

Rondal JA (1994b) Exceptional language development in mental retardation: Natural experiments in language modularity. Current Psychology of Cognition 13: 427–67.

Rondal JA (1995) Exceptional language development in Down syndrome. Implications for the cognition-language relationship. New York: Cambridge University Press.

Rondal JA (in press) Faire parler l'enfant retardé mental. un programme d'intervention psycholinguistique. Bruxelles: Labor.

Rondal JA and Comblain A (in press) Language in adults with Down syndrome in S Buckley (Ed) Language and cognitive development in Down's syndrome. London: Chapman and Hall.

Rondal JA and Edwards S (in press) Language in mental retardation. Acquisition, theory, and remediation. London: Whurr.

Rondal JA, Lambert JL and Sohier C (1981) Elicited verbal and nonverbal imitation in Down syndrome and other mentally retarded children : A replication and an extension of Berry. Language and Speech 24: 245–54.

Rosenberg S and Abbeduto L (1993) Language and communication in mental retardation. Development, processes, and intervention. Hillsdale N.J.: Erlbaum.

Ross M, Galaburda A and Kemper T (1984) Down's syndrome: Is there a decreased population of neurons? Neurology 34: 907–16.

Seagoe M (1965) Verbal development in a mongoloid. Exceptional children 6: 229–75.

Semmel E and Wiig E (1980) Clinical Evaluation of Language Functions (CELF). Columbus OH: Merrill.

Smith B and Oller K (1981) A comparative study of pre-meaningful vocalizations produced by normally developing and Down's syndrome infants. Journal of Speech and Hearing Disorders 46: 46–51.

Snyder-McLean L and McLean J (1987) Effectiveness of early intervention for children with language and communication disorders. In M Guralnick and F Bennett (Eds) The effectiveness of early intervention for at risk and handicapped children, pp.213–74. New York: Academic Press.

Sokolov J (1992) Linguistic imitation in children with Down syndrome. American Journal on Mental Retardation 97: 209–21.

Steffelaar J and Evenhuis H (1989) Life expectancy, Down syndrome, and dementia. Lancet: 492–3.

Sudhalter V, Scarborough H and Cohen I (1991) Syntactic delay and pragmatic deviance in the language of males with fragile X syndrome. American Journal of Medical Genetics 43: 65–71.

Vallar G and Papagno C (1993) Preserved vocabulary acquisition in Down's syndrome: The role of phonological short-term memory. Cortex 29: 467–83.

Vilkman E, Niemi J and Ikonen U (1988) Fragile X speech phonology in Finnish. Brain and Language 34: 203–21.

Wang P (1992 June) Relationship of neuropsychological and neurobiological profiles in Williams and Down syndromes. Paper presented at the Symposium 'Two genetic syndromes of contrasting cognitive profiles: A neuropsychological and neurobiological dissection' of the American Psychological Society, San Diego CA.

Wang P, Doherty S, Hesselink J and Bellugi U (1992) Callosal morphology concurs with neuropathological findings in two neurodevelopmental disorders. Archives of Neurology 49:407–11.

Wishart J (1988) Early learning in infants and young children with Down syndrome. In L Nadel (Ed) The psychobiology of Down syndrome, pp.7–50. Cambridge MA: MIT Press.

Wisniewski, K (1990) Down syndrome children often have brain with maturation delay, retardation of growth, and cortical dysgenesis. American Journal of Medical Genetics Supplement 7: 274–81.

Wisniewski K and Kida E (1994) Abnormal neurogenesis and synaptogenesis in Down syndrome brain. Developmental Brain Dysfunction 17: 1-12.

Wisniewski K, Laure-Kamionowska M, Connell F and Wen G (1986) Neuronal density and synaptogenesis in the postnatal stage of brain maturation in Down syndrome. In C Epstein (Ed) The neurobiology of Down syndrome, pp.29–44. New York: Raven Press.

Yoder D and Miller J (1972) What we may know and what we can do: Input towards a system. In J McLean, D Yoder and R Schiefelbusch (Eds) Language intervention with the retarded: Developing strategies, pp.89–107. Baltimore: University Park Press.

Zisk P and Bialer I. (1967) Speech and language problems in mongolism: A review of the literature. Journal of Speech and Hearing Disorders 32: 228–41.

# 8
# The Practical and Theoretical Significance of Teaching Literacy Skills to Children with Down's Syndrome

SUE BUCKLEY, GILLIAN BIRD AND ANGELA BYRNE

## 8.1 Introduction

In our view, the benefits of learning to read for children with Down's syndrome (DS) go beyond simply acquiring a functionally useful level of reading and writing skill. We will argue that the majority of children with DS can learn to read and that progress in reading can also develop speech and language skills, auditory perceptual skills and working memory function – all areas where children with DS usually display difficulties (Fowler 1990; Hulme and Mackenzie 1992).

Drawing on the limited amount of published research on literacy that is currently available and our own experience of teaching children with DS (Buckley 1985; Buckley *et al.* 1993; Buckley and Bird 1993; Bird and Buckley 1994) this overview will therefore address four issues; the *levels of literacy* to be expected, appropriate *teaching methods*, the children's *reading strategies* and the benefits for other *cognitive skills.*

## 8.2 What Levels of Literacy Skills can we Expect Children with Down's Syndrome to Achieve?

At the present time, it is not possible to give an accurate answer to this question. Reading is a skill that needs to be taught, and until all children with DS have access to appropriate literacy teaching, it is not possible to determine what proportion of the population can achieve a functional level of literacy nor the range of achievement that may be possible. However a review of the existing data may give some indications to guide parents and educators and serve as a baseline against which future achievements can be compared.

Two studies published in the UK in the 1980s indicate very limited reading progress in the first years at school. Casey *et al.* (1988) followed the progress of 36 children with DS, 18 in mainstream placements and 18 in schools for children with moderate learning difficulties. The children did not differ in cognitive development at the start of their schooling. After two years, 90% of the girls and 67% of the boys in the mainstream classrooms could achieve scores on both the accuracy and the comprehension components of the *Neale Reading Test*. The children in the special schools were lagging behind, with 90% of the girls and 33% of the boys scoring on accuracy, and only 44% of the girls and 33% of the boys scoring on comprehension. As the children were equally able at the start of the study, it is likely that the difference in reading progress two years later is due to differences in the teaching of reading in the two school types.

In a study of 58 children with DS in Manchester, Lorenz *et al.* (1985) report that at 5 years of age 47% of the children could read their own name and 19% read 5–10 words, at 6 years the figures for these two levels of attainment were 63% and 32%, at 7 years, 75% and 44%. In a survey of 90 teenagers in the UK (Buckley and Sacks 1987) parents reported that 66 of the teenagers could read at least a 'social–sight' vocabulary. Of these 66 readers, just half could read more than 50 words and 15 (16% of the total group) could be described as quite good readers who enjoyed reading books, including adventure stories and books on sport or nature. In this study, many parents commented that their teenagers attempted to master the TV, sport and pop pages of the newspaper and that even those unable to read, enjoyed looking at books and being read to. Carr and Hewitt (1982), reporting on a group of 43 16-year-olds, state that seven could read quite well, about the same proportion of the group as that in the Buckley and Sacks study. The reader is reminded that the data from all these surveys are difficult to interpret as many of the children included in the study will not have been taught to read at all. We certainly cannot assume that all the children and young people had reached the upper limit of their reading ability.

## 8.3 Individual Case Studies

The functional literacy skills of individual children with DS were being reported as early as 1961 by Butterfield and 1964 by Seagoe. The young men described in these papers had been taught by their parents as had Nigel Hunt, who had his diary, *The World of Nigel Hunt,* published in 1966. The foreword to this book, written by Nigel's father, describes the difficulties he experienced when trying to convince the educators of the time that Nigel could actually read and write!

It was the progress of Sarah Duffen as described by her father Leslie that first drew our attention to the possibility that children with DS could achieve functional levels of literacy and that reading might accelerate speech and language acquisition (Duffen 1976). Sarah's progress suggested that it might be valuable to start teaching children to read from as early as two or three years of age. Since 1981, we have been exploring this approach and have accumulated a number of case studies of which the following are examples of early readers who continued to have good teaching.

Daniel was introduced to reading at 2 years 4 months when he had a production vocabulary of about 50 single words. He learned to read 10 words in two months and these were chosen to build two-word phrases for him to read at 2 years 8 months. These were rapidly transferred to his speech, according to the observations recorded by his home-visiting teacher (Norris 1989). By 2 years 11 months Daniel was reading six three-word phrases, which again he rapidly began to use in his speech. At 3 years 4 months he could read 66 flashcards and many two and three-word combinations of these. The next month he was reading simple books and the words 'and' and 'a' appeared in his speech. At 3 years 6 months he was reading four-word sentences and at 3 years 8 months he could read 116 words and was speaking in six-word sentences. Daniel's rapid progress continued and, at 8 years of age, his reading age was 12 years 4 months and spelling age 9 years 9 months on the school assessment. Daniel finds handwriting difficult.He is still printing and prefers to use a word-processor for writing. He reads punctuation correctly but leaves much of it out when writing. He is being educated in a mainstream school and is average in his class for all subjects.

Louise was introduced to reading at 3 years 2 months when she learned to read her family names, 'Mummy', 'Daddy', 'Stephen' and 'Louise' by playing matching games. Two months later, she learned 'car', 'book', 'shoe', 'teddy', 'ball' and 'dolly'. At 3 years 7 months 'walking', 'sleeping' and 'drinking' were added and she read two-word phrases such as 'Louise walking', 'Mummy sleeping'. Louise's mother and the speech and language therapist worked together, making simple books and a dictionary of pictures into which Louise had to slot the words in the right pages. At 4 years 4 months she could read 35 single words on flashcards and some two-word sentences. She could also pick out known words in storybooks. Two months later, she could read more than 60 words and short phrases, in games, in full sentences and in books. She was also able to memorize and say whole sentences that she had previously read. Louise is now 8 years 8 months and has a reading accuracy age of 7 years 4 months and a reading comprehension age of 6 years 8 months on the *Neale Reading Test*. She is progressing well with both reading and writing, forming capitals as well as lower-case letters in joined handwriting.

Alistair learned to read in the same way as Daniel and Louise. At 10 years 8 months he has a reading accuracy age of 7 years 11 months and a comprehension age of 6 years 9 months on the Neale test. These three children are typical of those that we work with. Writing and spelling progress shows considerable variation among the children. In the UK the children begin to have spellings to learn and spelling tests from their third year in school at age 7 years. Our observations indicate that, early on, the children are 'visual' spellers. For example, Catherine's teacher reports that at 6 years she writes the word, looks at it to see if it looks right and if not corrects it. At 7 years, Daniel was still a 'visual' speller but at 9 years is a 'phonic' speller. While case studies such as these are valuable, they do not allow us to generalize about the potential for literacy for all children with DS. The children described have benefited from early intervention at home, continuous teaching from their parents, and mainstream schooling. We have worked with other children who made the same preschool progress but who received no further literacy teaching in their special schools, so can read no more as teenagers than they could as 5-year-olds. In order to advance our understanding, we need to be able to study representative population samples of children with DS longitudinally, collecting the same data on all the children and keeping detailed records of the teaching that they are receiving. With one of our graduate students, we have just embarked on such a study (Byrne *et al.* 1995). We are following the progress of 24 children with DS (age range 5–10 years at the outset) and comparing their progress with a group of their mainstream classmates who are matched with them on reading age, as well as classmates who are average readers for their age.

The study will chart the reading, writing and spelling progress of the children, look at the cognitive strategies they are using to read and the links between reading, language and memory skills. All the children with DS are learning to read and their reading ages range from 5 years to 8 years 5 months at the start of the study. The children with DS, while matched with the slower readers on the reading measures, are significantly behind them on the number, language and memory measures. In other words, the children with DS show advanced reading ability compared with all their other cognitive skills at this time. All the cognitive measures illustrate steady progress with age for the children with DS, though it must be remembered that these are cross-sectional not longitudinal data. We are collecting longitudinal data for all these 24 children, so will be able to report on the range of individual profiles of progress in due course.

## 8.4 How Should They be Taught to Read and Write?

In addressing the question of teaching methods, the relevant issue is whether there are any differences in the way one should teach a child with DS to read compared with the teaching methods used for typically-developing children. In our view, the same methods should be used for all children but teachers will need to take account of the relative delay in language knowledge and memory skills of the children with DS when teaching them to read.

We would teach all children by establishing a small sight vocabulary first, choosing words and sentences that the children use everyday in their speech and encouraging them to build their own phrases and sentences with this sight vocabulary. Next, while continuing to expand their sight vocabulary, we would be teach letter-sound correspondences – this using the words the children can already read in order to show them, from the start, how the letter-sound knowledge can help them to read an unfamiliar word. We would encourage the children to write from the start, tracing over words and sentences with fingers and pens, then moving on to copying and free writing. This approach fits in with the research on children's reading development which indicates that all children go from a *logographic stage* (when words are recognized by 'sight' only) to an *alphabetic stage* (when words can be 'sounded out' letter-by-letter) and then to an *orthographic stage* (Frith 1985; Gathercole and Baddeley 1993a). Frith emphasizes that it is the activity of writing and spelling that develops the child's use of an alphabetic strategy.

## 8.5 Three Reading Strategies

The research shows that there are three strategies that can be used when reading, 'visual', 'phonological' and 'context'. Firstly, as printed words become familiar to the reader, they are stored in a visual word store in the brain and are then recognized directly, when reading, by comparison with the stored visual image. This is called the 'direct visual' route for reading. Secondly, once letter-sound rules are known, then an unfamiliar word can be read by 'sounding it out' to identify its spoken form using the store of spoken word forms that have been established in the brain during learning to talk. This is called the 'phonological' route to reading. When faced with an unfamiliar word in a sentence, a third strategy for encoding it can be used, that of 'context'. The word can be guessed as one which will be grammatically correct and fit the story. Here the reader is drawing on their language knowledge to find the word rather than decoding it visually or phonologically. In reality, more than one strategy may be in use simultaneously. For example, if using context to guess an unfamiliar word in a sentence, several words might fit in semantically and grammatically, but only one of these synonyms will match the letters on the page phonically, so a final correct choice will depend on letter-sound knowledge. Young children at the logographic stage, with little phonic knowledge, may be quite happy to guess and insert a word that is semantically correct, but not orthographically correct, so might, for example, read 'shut' when the printed word is 'closed' (Buckley 1985; Seymour and Elder 1986).

Children with DS often seem to be good 'visual' readers, finding it relatively easy to establish a sight vocabulary from as early as two years of age. Using the phonological route and the context strategy depends on any child having an adequate knowledge of vocabulary and grammar. The word can only be decoded by 'sounding out' if the word is in the child's spoken vocabulary. A word can only be guessed as the one that will fit in the sentence if it is a known word and if the child is able to understand the whole sentence, both syntactically and semantically. This will require the sentence structure to be at a grammatical level that the child has mastered, and even then the ideas conveyed will only be understood if they are within the child's experience. Children with DS will usually have considerably less language knowledge than other children at their reading level, so be less able to use context and phonological decoding strategies to access words and meaning. Further, to be good at phonological decoding, a child must be able to hear all the sounds in the words and, given the hearing loss and auditory processing problems that children with DS often have, they are likely to be less able to use this route with ease than their typically developing peers. Our observations however, suggest that despite these very real additional difficulties experienced by the child with DS compared with typically-developing children, they *do* progress to being able to use phonological decoding for reading and spelling and they *are* able to use context. For the teacher, it is essential that they understand the level of skills that a child brings to the task and that they help the child to progress slowly but steadily in using all three strategies. It is particularly important that teachers know how much language knowledge a child has in order to avoid exposing the child to material that he or she can read aloud but cannot decode for meaning. Further, all children learn new language from reading so it is very important that the teacher appreciates that reading can be a powerful way to help children to expand their language knowledge (Garton and Pratt 1989). Evidence presented in the case histories and later in this chapter suggests that learning new language from reading may be more effective for the child with DS than learning from listening, as they have significant auditory processing and memory difficulties which visual learning may help to overcome. Are they using the same cognitive strategies to read as other typically-developing peers?

Our observational data to date suggest that children with DS are using the same strategies as typically-developing children when learning to read, though they may progress from the logographic to the alphabetic stage rather more slowly. We have records of children making both visual errors (e.g. confusing 'this' and 'shoe' or 'hair' and 'rain') and semantic errors (e.g., reading 'closed' for 'shut' or 'flannel' for 'bath') characteristic of the logographic stage in the early stages of their reading development, when they have no knowledge of letter-sound rules. Later they progress to an alphabetic stage and are able to use phonic knowledge for reading and spelling. As their vocabulary and knowledge of grammar grows, they are increasingly able to use context to identify new words.

Our longitudinal study will provide more adequate information as we are assessing their strategy use and progress over time using a variety of computerized tasks based on Seymour and Elder (1986).

## 8.6 Will the Activity of Learning to Read Develop Other Cognitive Skills?

Research on the links between typically-developing children's reading progress and other aspects of cognitive development suggest reciprocal interactions. The more language knowledge and the better the phonological awareness and working memory skills children bring to the task of reading, the faster they will learn to read in the first year of reading instruction. In the second year, reading success appears to develop working memory and phonological awareness skills (Ellis and Large 1988; Gathercole and Baddeley 1993b). Being able to read opens up access to knowledge and the biggest vocabulary explosion for children is between the ages of about 7 and 16, when children are typically learning on average 3000 words every year (Nagy and Herman 1987). Reading and writing also teach children correct grammar (Hutt 1981).

While we are as yet unable to support the argument that progress in reading will have the same benefits for children with DS with sufficient data, the cross-sectional data that we have suggest that significant gains in reading scores, in digit span scores (a working memory measure) and in language measures occur over the same period (Byrne *et al.* 1995). This is suggestive of functional links between the abilities measured but of course cannot demonstrate the direction of any possible causal links. It is hoped that the longitudinal data on these children will increase our understanding of the issues and allow us to demonstrate the direction of the effects. We would contend that these skills, reading, language and working memory, are likely to be reciprocally interactive and that progress in any one may 'bootstrap' progress in another. In children with specific learning difficulties such as the children with DS the direction of this 'bootstrapping' between skills may not be the same at any one developmental point as that seen in typically-developing children.

One area where we do have some data is on the effect of reading on speech and language skills. For the young children, case study records suggest that reading encourages progress to longer utterances and improved grammar in speech. They also suggest that reading improves articulation and speech intelligibility. For most children with DS, there is a well documented lag between comprehension and expressive speech skills, probably due to a variety of difficulties which may include problems with word retrieval, sentence structuring and speech-motor control. The limited development of working memory may also be implicated so that reading may provide the opportunity to practise saying sentences which the child is unable to generate spontaneously even though he or she understands them. This hypothesis is supported by the results of work with adolescents with DS (Buckley 1993a, 1994, in press). In a study designed to improve the productive syntax of a group of 12 teenagers, teaching which used print to support the learning was more effective in teaching correct production over six different sentence structures than speech and picture-only teaching. All the teenagers did better in the reading condition (see Buckley 1993b), but there were large individual differences. The teenagers who gained the most were those with no reading ability and the smallest digit spans. At the end of the training year, the teenagers demonstrated a significant gain in comprehension of grammar compared with a previous baseline year of no intervention beyond ordinary school practice and a significant increase in the length of the utterances that they used in everyday conversation (Buckley 1995).

## 8.8 Conclusion

We hope that we have convinced the reader that most children with DS are able to achieve a useful level of literacy ability and that all the children should have an opportunity to learn to read, as even a small sight vocabulary will help their speech and language skills and may improve their auditory discrimination and working memory function. Reading instruction should be considered as soon as the child has single word comprehension as the earlier the child is able to establish a sight vocabulary, the greater the benefit for his or her language and cognitive development.

## Acknowledgements

The authors would like to express their thanks to all the schools, parents and children without whom this work would not have been possible.

## References

Bird G Buckley SJ and (1994) Meeting the educational needs of children with Down's syndrome. Portsmouth UK, University of Portsmouth (ISBN 1-898-108-27-7).

Buckley SJ (1985) Attaining basic educational skills: reading, writing and number. In D Lane and B Stratford (Eds) Current approaches to Down's Syndrome, pp. 315–43. London: Cassell.

Buckley SJ (1993b) Developing the speech and language skills of teenagers with Down's syndrome. Down's Syndrome: Research and Practice 1(2): 63–71.

Buckley SJ (1993a) Improving the expressive grammar of teenagers with Down's syndrome. In J Clibbens and B Pendleton (Eds) Proceedings of the Child Language Seminar 281–9. Plymouth UK: University of Plymouth.

Buckley SJ (in press) Increasing the conversational utterance length of teenagers with Down's syndrome. Down's Syndrome: Research and Practice.

Buckley SJ and Bird G (1993) Teaching children with Down's syndrome to read. Down's Syndrome: Research and Practice 1: 34–41.

Buckley SJ, Emslie M, Haslegrave G and Le Prevost P (1993) The development of language and reading skills in children with Down's syndrome. Portsmouth UK: Portsmouth Polytechnic.

Buckley SJ and Sacks BI (1987) The adolescent with Down's syndrome – life for the teenager and for the family. Portsmouth UK, Portsmouth Polytechnic (ISBN: 0-900234-19-9).

Butterfield EC (1961) A provocative case of overachievement by a mongoloid. American Journal of Mental Deficiency 66: 444–8.

Byrne A, Buckley S, MacDonald J and Bird G (1995) Investigating the literacy, language and memory skills of children with Down's syndrome. Down's Syndrome: Research and Practice 3(2): 53–58.

Carr J and Hewitt S (1982) Children with Down's syndrome growing up. Child Psychology and Psychiatry News 10: 10–13.

Casey W, Jones D, Kugler B and Watkins B (1988) Integration of Down's syndrome children in the primary school: a longitudinal study of cognitive development and academic attainments. British Journal of Educational Psychology 58: 279–86.

Duffen L (1976) Teaching reading to teach language. Remedial Education 11: 139–42.

Ellis N and Large B (1988) The early stages of reading: A longitudinal study. Applied Cognitive Psychology 2: 47–76.

Fowler A (1990) Language abilities in children with Down syndrome: evidence for specific syntactic delay. In D Cicchetti and M Beeghly (Eds) Children with Down syndrome: A developmental perspective, pp. 302–43. New York: Cambridge University Press.

Frith U (1985) Beneath the surface of developmental dyslexia. In KE Patterson, JC Marshall and M Coltheart (Eds) Surface dyslexia 301–34. Hove UK: Erlbaum.

Gathercole S and Baddeley A (1993a) Working memory and language. Hove UK: Erlbaum.

Gathercole S and Baddeley A (1993b) Phonological working memory: A critical building block for reading development and vocabulary acquisition. European Journal of the Psychology of Education 8: 259–72.

Garton A and Pratt C (1989) Learning to be literate. Oxford UK: Blackwell.

Hulme C and MacKenzie S (1992) Working memory and severe learning difficulty. Hove UK: Erlbaum.

Hunt N (1966) The World of Nigel Hunt. London: Darwen Finlayson.

Hutt EL (1981) Teaching Language Disordered Children: A structured curriculum. London: Arnold.

Lorenz S, Sloper P and Cunningham C (1985) Reading and Down's syndrome. British Journal of Special Education 13: 65–7.

Nagy WE and Herman PA (1987) Breadth and depth of vocabulary knowledge: implications for acquisition and instruction. In MG McKeown and ME Curtis (Eds) The nature of vocabulary acquisition, pp. 19–35. Hillsdale NJ: Erlbaum.

Norris H (1989 April) Teaching reading to help develop language in very young children with Down's syndrome. Paper presented at the National Portage Conference, Peterborough UK.

Seagoe MV (1964) Yesterday was Tuesday, all day and all night: The story of a unique education. Toronto: Little Brown.

Seymour PHK and Elder L (1986) Beginning reading without phonology. Cognitive Neuropsychology 3: 1–36.

# 9 Alternative and Augmentative Systems of Communication for Children with Down's Syndrome

BOB REMINGTON AND SUE CLARKE

## 9.1 Introduction

Many children with Down's syndrome (DS) experience severe language delay. To gain some insight into what this must be like, to understand its impact on development, and to think about the importance of language intervention, it is worth briefly considering an analogy. Recall how it feels to arrive in a foreign country whose language is unfamiliar; such conditions can rapidly lead to feelings of isolation, helplessness, stupidity and defeat.

Fortunately, there are some things that can be done to overcome a communication barrier such as this even before beginning to speak a new language. For example, the use of primitive gestures – such as pointing, leading, many facial expressions – is usually a relatively transparent way of communicating across cultures and therefore immediately effective. At a slightly more sophisticated level, some manual signs may be used to facilitate communication. Drinking can be mimed by bringing a cupped hand to the mouth, walking by flexing downward-pointed fingers, and so on. Some signs have a more abstract quality – the thumbs up sign meaning 'okay' for example. However, the meanings of many such signs are based on cultural convention, and therefore are not universally understood. Finally, visual symbols can be used to effect communication, for example by pointing to (or even drawing) a picture; writing or pointing to text.

As well as helping the unilingual traveller, all of these means of communication can help the person with mental retardation who has not yet acquired a first language. Research on the educational and clinical use of gestures, signs and symbols for communicative purposes is studied under the generic name of Alternative and Augmentative Communication (AAC). There is already a growing body of empirical literature and an international journal, *Augmentative and Alternative Communication*, devoted since 1985 to work in this area. The aim of this chapter is to discuss the relevance of AAC to the education of children with DS.

A speaker in a foreign country who needs to acquire a second language is, of course, in many ways very different from a child who has yet to acquire a first language; the comparison should not be taken too far. Nevertheless, there are sufficient similarities at the level of communication difficulties to make it worthwhile to use the analogy to evaluate the potential benefits of AAC.

In what might be seen as the 'worst case scenario', sign- or symbol-based communication can serve as a genuine alternative to speech for both the hapless traveller and the language-delayed child. Provided that the messages to be communicated are very simple, and that the communication situations are familiar, rudimentary forms of AAC can be quite effective. For children who, in addition to mental retardation, experience extreme articulatory problems or profound hearing impairments that render speech acquisition particularly difficult, AAC is certainly a viable option. As we will see later, some of the more sophisticated forms of sign- or symbol-based communication may be considered to have many, or all, the properties of spoken languages. For most travellers and most children with mental retardation, however, this degree of sophistication will not be relevant. For them, signs, symbols and gestures act as a supplement to speech. They may aid communication in situations where a simple vocabulary and elementary knowledge of syntax is not quite enough to get by. And, in the course of supplementing speech, AAC may serve a third function – that of providing a gateway to speech. There are a number of reasons why a supplementary means of communication may eventually facilitate speech acquisition, either as a second language or as a first.

Speech normally offers the most effective method of controlling socially mediated outcomes; unilingual travellers, and children with severe language delay, have no access to this means of control. Research has consistently shown that under any conditions where such important outcomes cannot be controlled, a state of 'learned helplessness' – an amotivational syndrome akin to depression – may ensue (Seligman 1975). However, because speech and AAC may be seen as different forms of verbal behaviour with functionally equivalent effects (Skinner 1957), AAC may provide a means of controlling the social environment that can be maintained even in the absence of normal speech development. Thus AAC teaching can reduce helplessness and may, moreover, be positively motivation-enhancing in that it provides a medium through which efforts to communicate can be regularly reinforced. By the same token, effective communication by a learner reinforces the teaching of AAC, essentially creating 'a virtuous circle' of increased interaction and communication. This blossoming level of social activity can provide a further route to speech acquisition by ensuring that the sounds of language are heard in just the meaningful contexts necessary to facilitate understanding – a pathway to immersion. AAC thus helps to make clear to others where help is needed, and what needs to be learned.

Finally, there is substantial evidence that the self-injury, aggression and other forms of 'challenging' behaviours sometimes seen in individuals with severe mental retardation can function communicatively: that is, such behaviours can have functionally equivalent properties to requests for attention or demand reduction (Carr and Durand 1985; Durand and Crimmins 1991; Remington 1993). This interpretation is based on evidence that these behaviours can be reduced by displacing them with verbal requests, based either on speech or on AAC (Carr and Durand 1985; Duker and Remington 1991).

To summarize, AAC has three distinguishable roles in facilitating effective communication. First, it can provide a substitute for speech in children with little possibility of acquiring vocal fluency. Second, in children whose language is delayed, it can provide a supplement to the speech that they have already learned. Finally, AAC can create a pathway to speech by reducing helplessness, enhancing the motivation of both the teachers and the pupil, creating clear communication contexts for interpreting the sounds of speech, and – in the case of some children with severe mental retardation – reducing challenging behaviours that may interfere with effective language acquisition. Before considering the particular benefits of AAC for children with DS, we will briefly review the kinds of AAC systems that have been studied.

## 9.2 Types of AAC System

The most familiar forms of AAC are manual sign languages such as American or British Sign Language (ASL and BSL) used by people with hearing impairments. Such systems have been shown to have many of the functional and structural characteristics of spoken language (Klima and Bellugi 1979), but simplified versions are normally taught to children experiencing language delays. One such system, Makaton (Walker 1978), is based on BSL and is widely used in the UK. A number of visual symbol vocabularies have also been developed, mainly based on pictographic symbols (see Vanderheiden and Lloyd 1986, for a review). These include Picsyms, PCS and Makaton symbols. Some more abstract symbols are also available, notably Blissymbols (Silverman *et al.* 1978), a system based on combining visual units with elementary semantic content to make more complex semantic units.

The diversity of systems available and in use reflects a range of historical origins. Ultimately, the potential benefits of intervention with any of these systems will be evaluated empirically, but as yet there are relatively few well-controlled studies. Nevertheless, it is possible to compare the strengths and weaknesses of gestural (sign-based) and graphic (symbol-based) modes of AAC at a conceptual level on a number of dimensions.

Signs and symbols differ primarily in terms of the process for producing utterances. Like speech sounds, manual signs must be manufactured by generating motorically complex handshapes with varying levels of performance difficulty (e.g., one-handed *vs.* two-handed signs; identical *vs.* non-identical left and right hand movements, etc.), whereas symbols are 'activated' by the simple act of pointing. Thus, symbols are normally recognized and chosen from an array provided by a teacher, whereas manual signs must be actively recalled and, literally, manufactured. It also follows from these cognitive and motoric considerations that signing is relatively harder to prompt than symbol use, and that, through difficulties in execution, signs are less likely to be clearly interpretable. Comprehension processes differ to the extent that in complex 'utterances' the manual signs may be transient, as one handshape replaces another. By comparison, symbols are more easily interpreted if they can be placed to make a message in such a way that they can be repeatedly scanned.

Other considerations reflect how well the different kinds of systems can be used to interact with individuals who are unfamiliar with them. Here, symbol systems have some substantial advantages. First, they are generally more iconic than signs. Iconicity is operationalized as translucency or transparency where transparency refers to ease of guessing, and translucency to the degree to which the sign 'makes sense' once its meaning is revealed (e.g. the sign for 'red' consists of touching one's lips). Symbols are typically pictographic, so their meaning is transparent, but sign meanings are more often merely translucent or conventional. Signs are apparently superior in terms of usability by comparison with symbols, for the latter always require some physical medium on which to appear, for example a series of flash cards, a communication board (i.e., a large matrix display), or a computer screen. But the level of inconvenience related to symbol systems is rapidly declining with the advent of small hand-held communication aids, and modern systems have some compensating benefits, most importantly the capacity to produce an immediately comprehensible vocal message from a tape or speech synthesizer. The fact that symbols can now be used to generate communicative speech (and that their meaning can anyway be clarified by written labels) makes most symbols easier for non-users to understand than all but the simplest signs.

These comparisons raise the issue of choice – which AAC system is most appropriate for children with DS? But first we must consider the more basic question: is AAC in principle an appropriate method for language intervention with such children? In the sections which follow we argue that AAC is indeed useful in this context, and can in fact provide particular benefits which compensate for some of the most commonly identified difficulties in language acquisition experienced by children with DS.

## 9.3 Is AAC Appropriate for Children with Down's Syndrome?

The critical issue which underlies this question concerns whether learning an AAC system could undermine or otherwise impede progress towards oral language, an argument familiar to those who have worked with hearing impairment. If a child has a serious hearing or speech production problem, recommending AAC is less problematic, but for other children the impact of AAC on speech needs examination. As the 'unilingual traveller' analogy suggests, there are some very strong intuitive reasons for rejecting the view that a non-vocal system will interfere with the subsequent learning of speech. Rather, at a general level AAC intervention may provide a gateway to speech by locking a child more firmly into the social world as an actor. Empirically, several experimental studies show that, for imitative children at least, functional speech can be directly attributed to sign training (Carr and Dores 1981; Remington and Clarke 1983) and several case studies indicate that sign or symbol training is associated with speech gains.

There may still be some residual concerns that, once a limited but effective vocabulary has been learned, the motivation for going further can fall away. There is no reason in principle why this should happen, any more than we would expect mainstream children to stop at a one-word vocabulary, but clearly this concern must be on a teacher's agenda – if the aim of teaching is merely to produce an AAC vocabulary, benefits are likely to be limited. At this point it is important to emphasize that using an AAC system does not plunge the child into a silent world where speech is taboo. As we will see, AAC systems are typically used in parallel with speech, the method known as simultaneous (or 'total') communication. For teachers and parents, AAC therefore serves augmenting and clarifying functions, marking particular spoken words with an emphasis that would otherwise not be possible. For children who are not effective verbally – as a result of either overall delay or specific articulatory problems – AAC offers another channel through which to enter the social world and control it directly and relatively effortlessly.

We can conclude that some form of AAC is very likely to be appropriate whenever a child is experiencing a significant language delay. A policy of zero exclusion from AAC is advocated by some (e.g., Baumgart *et al.* 1990) and this position is reasonable provided that the acquisition of single-sign or symbol vocabulary is not seen as an end in itself. It is essential that parents and teachers take advantage of the gateway to speech that AAC provides.

Turning now to the role of AAC for children with DS, Buckley (1993) has recently provided a highly pertinent analysis of their language development. Her main conclusions (p.7) can be briefly paraphrased thus:

Children with Down's syndrome may:

1. from infancy, experience hearing loss, visual defects and motor delay which impedes their progress;
2. as toddlers, be slower at learning new words and expanding their total vocabulary and slower than expected in terms of their progress measured by MA;
3. from infancy, experience differences in the way mothers talk to them that could adversely affect progress;
4. show specific productive delays; their comprehension for vocabulary and syntax usually exceeds productive skill;
5. have more difficulty in learning grammar and syntax than lexical items;
6. have difficulty speaking clearly, showing both phonological and articulatory difficulties.

We have made use of many of Buckley's descriptive phrases in the tabulation above, primarily to indicate how close the match is between the difficulties experienced by children with DS and the potential benefits for remediation offered by AAC systems. Considering each item in turn:

1. For DS children with hearing loss, AAC can exploit the visual communication channel, and only the most severe forms of motor delay interfere with symbol acquisition. Although sign learning requires effective motor control, signs – unlike vocal utterances – can be physically prompted by moulding the hands appropriately.
2. The idea of using AAC systems to remediate the delay in vocabulary acquisition is very promising because, compared with their spoken equivalents, single signs or symbols are non-evanescent, often iconic, easier to imitate or prompt, and easier to remember.
3. The relatively low levels of appropriate 'conversational' behaviour in DS infants and toddlers may be remediated by encouraging parents consciously to structure their interactions. AAC provides a useful medium for this approach because the learning situation is inherently more structured. Specifically, teaching procedures focus joint atten-

tion on visual signs or symbols and referents, and conversational roles are thus more clearly marked.

4. As indicated earlier, AAC simplifies production processes dramatically, and there is some evidence (see below) that its acquisition is facilitated by an existing understanding of speech (Clarke *et al.* 1986, 1988; Light *et al.* 1989; Romski and Sevcik 1993).
5. Problems in the initial acquisition of syntax may be facilitated by the use of AAC methods which can mark syntactic relations very clearly (Light *et al.* 1990). Non-evanescent symbols may be particularly useful in this context because they lend themselves to highly structured ways of teaching syntactic strings (Carrier and Peak 1975).
6. AAC can compensate for phonological and articulatory difficulties, disambiguating difficult-to-understand speech by allowing children the opportunity to communicate in parallel through auditory and visual channels.

To summarize, in virtually all the particulars where children with DS have problems, signs and symbols can provide solutions, either as an alternative to speech or as a way of augmenting and eventually developing it. This is all very good news, but if AAC is to be used, how should it be implemented?

## 9.4 How is AAC Implemented and What is its Impact?

There are a number of critical issues relating to underlying assumptions about the nature of AAC. First, should the principles that guide AAC implementation be based on a developmental (norm-based) or needs-based (pragmatic) model?

### 9.4.1 Developmental analysis

Most experts (e.g., Reichle *et al.* 1991) argue that normative developmental data, such as prerequisites for language, must be used cautiously as a guide for intervention with AAC. There are a number of reasons for this. First, there are differences between the way that AAC systems and spoken language are used. Because AAC is almost always heavily supplemented by speech (simultaneous communication), any parallels that might otherwise exist are reduced. Secondly, and more generally, there are qualitative differences in adaptive behaviour between older children with mental retardation and younger MA-matched mainstream children which are the product of their different experiences. Considerations such as this reduce the potential value of using normal language development milestones or processes as a guide to intervention.

On the other hand, if AAC is providing a gateway to spoken language, the assessment of children's competence against developmental norms seems reasonable. For example, some analyses have combined performance with speech and sign to arrive at an indicator of the impact of AAC on overall language development (e.g., Miller 1993).

Finally, the developmental approach may be useful as a tool for reflecting on the development of communication using an AAC system (Gerber and Kraat 1992). The Makaton system (Walker 1978) seems to be based on this kind of developmental perspective, at least in so far as it is recommended that eight groups of Makaton vocabulary items are taught in a fixed order of 'stages' (Grove and Walker 1990, p.17). Unfortunately, some problems with the rigidity of this staged approach are immediately apparent (e.g., 'ball' is a stage 2 word; 'throw' a stage 5 word; ) and it has frequently been criticized (Byler 1985; Kiernan *et al.* 1982). Moreover, there are theoretical reasons for questioning the very idea of a vocabulary, at least during the early stages of acquisition of AAC. For example, signs or words learned to subserve one language function (e.g., requesting) do not automatically transfer to subserve another (e.g., commenting) (Goodman and Remington 1991; Lamarre and Holland 1985). A functionally based approach suggests a more effective way of implementing AAC interventions should be based on the situationally-determined individual communicative needs of children identified through a procedure known as *ecological analysis*.

### 9.4.2 Ecological analysis

Reichle *et al.* (1991) conceptualize communication not as a capacity that children have but as something that they do – a pattern of behaviour. A child's need to communicate is thus a product of his or her everyday environmental context, rather than some unfolding developmental timetable. This pragmatic, or functional, approach to language leads Reichle *et al.* to suggest that, before any AAC intervention begins, the circumstances of the learners should be analysed in detail, and intervention based on an understanding of their needs.

Analysis initially focuses on children's reasons for communication and attempts to identify how their communication needs are currently being met. Children may not communicate in a barren or undemanding environment and, as indicated earlier, various forms of non-vocal behaviour may be identified which serve communicative functions (Carr and Durand 1985). It is only when these preliminaries are known that to-be-taught communicative functions and necessary vocabulary can be identified, following which a decision can be made on the particular kind of AAC system most suited to a child's needs. The kinds of technical consideration on which this choice can be based have already been described above. The critical point to emphasize here is that this choice is made on the basis of an individualized analysis, such that the AAC system is matched to the needs of the particular child under consideration (Kiernan *et al.* 1982; Baumgart *et al.* 1990). Thus, it would be inappropriate to choose signs over symbols, or vice versa, on the basis of some kind of normative evaluation. The keynote in work of this kind is flexibility. Thus, there is no assumption that either signs or symbols must be used, and it is quite possible that a mixed system might be most appropriate for a particular child.

To summarize, practitioners of AAC should always consider the possibilities of an individually-tailored approach to intervention – not simply an off-the-peg package that takes no account of the needs of the communicator.

### 9.4.3 Naturalistic teaching approaches

The ecological approach leads more naturally to long-term intervention in everyday contexts rather than formal experimentation. There are a number of examples of studies of this kind – usually relying on uncontrolled single cases, and longitudinal in form. This type of research has substantial benefits in that it documents AAC and linguistic performance over time, revealing significant patterns of development. Its drawback is that the relative lack of control inherent in naturalistic work makes it harder, unambiguously, to attribute behavioural changes to intervention methods (Remington 1991). We will review some single case studies in this area before moving on to consider briefly some more controlled AAC intervention studies.

Layton and Savino (1990) worked with Bobby, a child with DS aged 2 years 10 months over a period of two years. Bobby's oral speech skills, including oral-motor control, vocal imitation and vocal initiation, were poor, despite normal hearing, and his mother considered that 'he had no way of communicating'. Intervention for one term using speech-only methods had virtually no impact, at which point simultaneous speech-manual sign teaching was initiated. This was based on natural communication around shared activities, an approach that Layton and Savino describe as 'child oriented'. Over a period of five terms this produced dramatic improvements in signing, such that by the end of the intervention Bobby could use around 500 signs. More significantly, however, oral language training was resumed in the final term and his vocal skills developed to the point that he could say 43 words intelligibly. By the age of 7 years, a follow-up assessment showed that Bobby used oral speech exclusively, with a vocabulary extending to more than 700 words. In the absence of control procedures, Layton and Savino (1990) are clear that the changes seen cannot be attributed unambiguously to the intervention but they assert that 'if nothing else, Bobby's communication and language skills were enhanced by his early sign training'.

Kouri (1989), working with another virtually non-vocal child with DS aged 2 years 8 months, has presented data that support this analysis. Over an 8-month intervention period, Kouri used a play-based procedure to introduce simultaneous speech-sign communication training and focused on the patterns of sign and word acquisition. The percentage of spoken productions increased in the second half of the intervention and the sign/simultaneous productions declined. This relative preference for speech with continued training was paralleled by a threefold increase in the absolute number of spoken productions from 276 to 745 words. It seems that, in naturalistic settings at least, signing in the context of simultaneous communication probably does not interfere with the acquisition of speech.

Similar conclusions can be drawn from work using symbol systems. For example, Pecyna (1988) carried out a similar case study using a rebus system with a child with DS. Romski and Sevcik (1993) provide a more comprehensive account of a larger, 2-year longitudinal study with 13 youths. Their average age was 12 years 4 months and they had spoken language impairments that were more severe than those of most children with DS (average receptive vocabulary age equivalent to 3 years 5 months and up to 10 intelligible words). These youths were given access to a computer based symbol system incorporating a speech synthesizer which allowed them to communicate in naturalistic settings using arbitrary symbols with English vocabulary attached. The use of the system was not forced; rather, teachers used a version of simultaneous communication in which normal speech paralleled symbol use with augmentation of key words (e.g., 'let's go *out* and play *ball*'). A regular schedule of assessment allowed teachers and parents to monitor progress carefully for the duration of the study. All learners acquired at least 20/30 symbols, with the most effective students rapidly learning very many more. There were improvements in printed word recognition, receptive speech and intelligible expressive speech. Moreover, these skills generalized to new partners and settings. A critical factor affecting how well the symbol system was acquired was the youth's pre-existing receptive language and communication skills, a finding paralleling our own on the role of receptive speech in facilitating the acquisition of expressive signing (Clarke *et al.* 1986, 1988). In some sense, Romski and Sevcik's participants extant knowledge of the vocal mode enhanced their acquisition of symbol use which in turn transcended their original capabilities in speech.

Finally, the recent work of Miller and his colleagues, based on a cross-sectional model, indicates that signing intervention can close the gap in language acquisition that appears between Down's syndrome and typically developing children (Miller 1993). Although there were significant differences between these groups on a speech-based measure of vocabulary, they could be removed by combining the speech- and sign-based vocabulary scores of the children with DS prior to making the comparison.

### 9.4.4 More formal teaching approaches

The work reviewed above emphasizes the practical benefits of a thoroughly naturalistic approach to teaching AAC to ensure that learning is functional and contextually appropriate. It has, however, been argued that a more structured form of teaching may sometimes be appropriate to teach language forms such as vocabulary items, and functions such as naming (Carr 1986; Clibbens 1993). The studies, which are briefly described below, were conducted at Southampton using teaching methods based on this more formal approach and, while the participants had severe language delays, they typically did not carry the diagnosis of Down's syndrome. However, we have every reason to believe that the implications of work of this kind are relevant in this context. One particular area where structured intervention may be useful is in managing the transition between single signs and sign combinations.

Remington *et al.* (1990) taught children to master attribute-object combinations to name coloured objects (e.g., 'red car', 'green cup'). Our method of teaching such combinations, which was designed to facilitate the emergence of untaught novel sign combinations, is called *matrix training*. If signs for colours are imagined as the rows of a two dimensional matrix, and signs for objects as the columns, it is possible to teach a sample of sign combinations corresponding to the cells lying on the stepped diagonal of the matrix, such that each object sign is taught with two colour signs and each colour sign with two object signs. Such training can then be followed by probes designed to test for the appearance of the novel – or productive – sign combinations which correspond to the outlying cells. In general, the amount of productivity following training in studies of this kind at Southampton was strongly affected by factors related to the children's prior knowledge of the stimulus items chosen for training. Children who, prior to matrix training, understood (but typically did not say) the colour and object names, and knew their corresponding signs, showed complete productivity throughout the matrix although only the diagonal items were explicitly trained. Furthermore, following training, these children could accurately combine single signs with which they were familiar but which they had never experienced as part of the matrix training procedure itself. It seems therefore that sign-combining skills can be built on skills with single signs, and these skills in turn are more easily acquired when the signs correspond to words in a child's receptive vocabulary as Clarke *et al.*'s (1986, 1988) and Romski and Sevcik's (1993) work has shown.

A matrix-based teaching procedure of the kind just described combines AAC elements semantically. In principle, however, there is no reason that it should not be extended to teach more basic syntactic relations (see Light *et al.* 1990 for discussion).

### 9.4.5 A hybrid teaching approach

A formal teaching procedure has the advantages that it allows control of complex teaching materials, and with a little ingenuity it can be adapted to naturalistic situations. For example, in recent work at Southampton, Hewitt (1995) used a school snack break as an opportunity to teach Dylan, a child with severe mental retardation, to combine pictographic colour-object symbols to request tableware. Dylan regularly helped to lay the table for the morning snack-break at his school. The 'rule' for place laying was that each child must have a cup, a plate, and a mat of a different colour. Thus, if a place setting was partly laid with – say – a red mat and a blue plate, Dylan was required to select a yellow cup. During request training, Hewitt controlled the tableware items available to Dylan, who learned to make requests for the hidden items using a colour-object symbol combination. The only combinations taught were those corresponding to the stepped diagonal of the colour-object matrix. Hewitt was able to show that this procedure was sufficient to produce productive generalization throughout the matrix, so that the child would spontaneously and appropriately request items using symbol combinations which had never been explicitly taught. This study is unusual in that it used a formal programme within a naturalistic setting, and contrived a situation in which the symbol combinations served a requesting rather than a commenting function.

Finally, because the requested table item was not visibly present, the use of the AAC symbol system had a spontaneous need-driven character to it: Dylan asked for what he wanted, even though he couldn't see it at the time he asked.

## 9.5 Conclusion: Does AAC Teaching Facilitate Language Development ?

Although little of the research in the area of AAC is as well controlled as the most rigorous methodologist would wish, the answer to this question seems to be a cautious 'yes'. For children who will never speak, AAC can provide an alternative to a world of silence and frustration. For many other children, AAC provides a gateway through to speech at the single word level, and for children who have already crossed that threshold, AAC may provide a step up to syntax. But equally, AAC acquisition itself may be based on what a child already knows about the social world in general, and the world of words in particular. There is a great deal more that we need to know about how AAC works. For example:

- How precisely does receptive speech mediate AAC acquisition?
- How does AAC acquisition affect other skills?

- How can we ensure spontaneity and conversational competence with AAC?
- How can we ensure children use AAC for the full range of pragmatic functions?
- How can we ensure productivity in AAC use?
- How can we best facilitate the transition between AAC and speech?

We have some kinds of answers to some of these questions, but there is much more to be learned. While research must continue, it is already clear that there are some quite overwhelming benefits to be had from the use of AAC in the education and development of children with Down's syndrome.

## References

Augmentative and Alternative Communication (1985) ISBN: 0743-4618. Baltimore MD: Williams and Wilkins.

Baumgart D, Johnson J and Helmstetter E (1990) Augmentative and alternative communication systems for persons with moderate and severe disabilities. Baltimore MD: Brookes.

Buckley S (1993) Language development in children with Down's syndrome: Reasons for optimism. Down's syndrome: Research and Practice 1: 3–9.

Byler J (1985) The Makaton vocabulary: An analysis based on recent research. British Journal of Special Education 12: 113–20.

Carr EG (1986) Behavioral approaches to language and communication. In E Schopler and G Mesibov (Eds) Current issues in autism Vol 3: Communication problems in autism, pp. 37–57. New York: Plenum Press.

Carr EG and Dores PA (1981) Patterns of language acquisition following simultaneous communication with autistic children. Analysis and Intervention in Developmental Disabilities 1: 347–61.

Carr EG and Durand VM (1985) Reducing behavior problems through functional communication training. Journal of Applied Behavior Analysis 18: 111–26.

Carrier JK and Peak T (1975) Non-speech Language Initiation Program. Lawrence KS: H&H Enterprises.

Clarke S, Remington B and Light P (1986) An evaluation of the relationship between receptive speech skills and expressive signing. Journal of Applied Behavior Analysis 19: 231–9.

Clarke S, Remington B and Light P (1988) The role of referential speech in sign learning by mentally retarded children: A comparison of total communication and sign-alone training. Journal of Applied Behavior Analysis 21: 419–26.

Clibbens J (1993) From theory to practice in child language development. Down's syndrome: Research and Practice 1: 101–6.

Duker P and Remington B (1991) Manual sign-based communication for individuals with severe or profound learning difficulties. In B Remington (Ed) The challenge of severe mental handicap: A behaviour analytic approach, pp.167–87. New York: Wiley .

Durand VM and Crimmins D (1991) Teaching functionally equivalent responses as an intervention for challenging behavior. In B Remington (Ed) The challenge of severe mental handicap: A behaviour analytic approach, pp. 71-95. New York: Wiley.

Gerber S and Kraat A (1992) Use of a developmental model of language acquisition: Application to children using AAC systems. Augmentative and Alternative Communication 8: 19–32.

Goodman J and Remington B (1991) Teaching communicative signing: Labelling, requesting and transfer of function. In B Remington (Ed) The challenge of severe mental handicap: A behaviour analytic approach, pp. 215–34. New York: Wiley.

Grove N and Walker M (1990) The Makaton vocabulary: Using manual signs and graphic symbols to develop interpersonal communication. Augmentative and Alternative Communication 6: 15–28.

Hewitt J (1995) Using matrix training procedures to develop spontaneous and functional symbol communication. Unpublished doctoral dissertation, University of Southampton UK.

Kiernan CC, Reid B and Jones L (1982) Signs and symbols: Use of non-vocal communication systems. Studies in Education No.11 University of London, Institute of Education.

Klima ES and Bellugi U (1979) The signs of language. Cambridge MA: Harvard University Press.

Kouri T (1989) How manual sign acquisition relates to the development of spoken language: A case study. Language, Speech and Hearing Services in Schools 20: 50-62.

Lamarre J and Holland JG (1985) The functional independence of mands and tacts. Journal of the Experimental Analysis of Behavior 43: 5–19.

Layton T and Savino MA (1990) Acquiring a communication system by sign and speech in a child with Down syndrome: A longitudinal investigation. Child Language Teaching and Therapy 6: 59–76.

Light P, Remington B, Clarke S and Watson J (1989) Signs of language? In I Leudar, M Beveridge and G Conti-Ramsden (Eds) Language and communication in the mentally handicapped, pp.56–79. London: Chapman and Hall.

Light P, Watson J and Remington B (1990) Beyond the single sign II: The significance of sign order in a matrix-based approach to teaching productive sign combinations. Mental Handicap Research 3: 161–78.

Miller JF (1993) Development of speech and language in children with Down Syndrome. In IT Lott and EE McCoy (Eds) Down syndrome: Advances in medical care, pp.39–50. New York: Wiley-Liss.

Pecyna PM (1988) Rebus symbol communication training with a severely handicapped preschool child: A case study. Language, Speech and Hearing Services in Schools 19: 128–43.

Reichle J, York J and Sigafoos J (1991) Implementing augmentative and alternative communication: Strategies for learners with severe disabilities. Baltimore MD: Brookes.

Remington B (1991) Why use single subject methods in AAC? In J Brodin and E Bjorck-Åkesson (Eds) Methodological issues in research in augmentative and alternative communication. Proceedings of the First International ISAAC Research Symposium in augmentative and alternative communication, pp.74–8. Stockholm: Swedish Handicap Institute.

Remington B (1993) Challenging behaviour in people with severe learning disabilities: Behaviour modification or behaviour analysis? In C Kiernan (Ed) Research to practice? Implications of research on the challenging behaviour of people with learning disability, pp.119–34. Clevedon UK: BILD.

Remington B and Clarke S (1983) Acquisition of expressive signing by autistic children: An evaluation of the relative effects of simultaneous communication and sign-alone training. Journal of Applied Behavior Analysis 16: 315–28.

Remington B, Watson J and Light P (1990) Beyond the single sign: A matrix-based approach to teaching productive sign combinations. Mental Handicap Research 3: 33–50.

Romski MA and Sevcik RA (1993) Language learning through augmented means. In AP Kaiser and DB Gray (Eds) Enhancing children's communication: Research foundations for intervention, pp.85–104. Baltimore MD: Brookes.

Seligman MEP (1975) Helplessness: On depression, development and death. San Fransisco CA: Freeman.

Silverman H, McNaughton S and Kates B (1978) Handbook of Blissymbolics. Toronto, Canada: Blissymbolics Communication Institute.

Skinner BF (1957) Verbal behavior. New York: Appleton-Century-Crofts.

Vanderheiden GC and Lloyd LL (1986) Overview. In S Blackstone (Ed) Augmentative communication: An introduction, pp.201–34. Rockville MD: American Association on Speech, Language and Hearing.

Walker M (1978) The Makaton vocabulary. In T Tebbs (Ed) Ways and Means, pp.172–83. Basingstoke UK: Globe Education.

# Part Four: Early Intervention

# 10
# Future Directions in Early Intervention for Children with Down's Syndrome

MICHAEL J GURALNICK

## 10.1 Introduction

Early intervention remains one of the most visible and potentially important enterprises in the field of developmental disabilities today. Grounded in sound developmental theory and supported by an often compelling logic, early intervention programmes for children with a wide range of disabilities as well as those at-risk for developmental problems have now achieved a reasonable level of political and scientific acceptance worldwide (Guralnick, in press).

Yet it is only relatively recently that our field has achieved the level of understanding of child development and disability, and identified the mechanisms through which biological and environmental factors exert their influence, to appreciate both the value and limits of early intervention programmes. Of special significance is our emerging appreciation not only of the impact that can be achieved on intellectual development, the most frequent target of early intervention for children with Down's syndrome (DS) as well as others with general developmental delays, but of the potential for influencing other complex and integrative developmental domains such as social competence.

Accordingly, in this chapter, I will attempt to characterize the value and effectiveness of early intervention for children with DS within a contemporary developmental framework. In so doing, I will discuss not simply the traditional emphasis on children's intellectual development but also their social development, especially social competence with peers. It is anticipated that, by adopting a broader developmental framework, emerging knowledge of the influence of motivation, social-cognition and family processes, for example, on various aspects of the development of children with DS will advance our field. It is this interplay between developmental knowledge and early intervention programmes that provides an innovative, yet realistic framework to guide future directions for research and practice.

## 10.2 Effects on Intellectual Development

Assessments of the course of children's development in the absence of systematic early intervention programmes have provided an important perspective for researchers. Findings for children manifesting various risk factors and those with established disabilities have consistently revealed that without participation in early intervention programmes, measured intellectual development gradually declines over the first few years of life. The magnitude of this decline, assessed in terms of effect size, is approximately one-half to three-quarters of a standard deviation. This phenomenon has been observed repeatedly for children at biological risk primarily due to prematurity/low birthweight (Brooks-Gunn *et al.* 1993; Liaw and Brooks-Gunn 1993; Rauh *et al.* 1988), those raised in disadvantaged circumstances (Campbell and Ramey 1994), and those with broadly-based developmental delays (Dunst *et al.* 1986). Even the course of motor development for children with cerebral palsy follows a similar pattern in the absence of comprehensive early intervention (Palmer *et al.* 1988).

Of importance, research reported in the 1970s consistently revealed a similar pattern of decline in assessed intellectual development for children with DS not experiencing early intervention (Carr 1970; Connolly 1978; Melyn and White 1973; Morgan 1979). Even a recent report from South Africa, in which early intervention programmes were not yet available, yielded a similar outcome (Neser *et al.* 1989). It should be pointed out that in the case of assessed intellectual development, declines observed during the first few months of life, up to perhaps 18 months of age, are to be expected, due primarily to the dependence, early on, of tests of general intelligence on motor skills, and the strong biological constraints that operate for that domain (Bendersky and Lewis 1994; Shonkoff *et al.* 1992). Accordingly, the initial and most rapid decline that occurs during the first 18 months of life may well reflect the transition from motor to more cognitive and language-based test items. However, the continued decline may reflect, to some extent, non-optimal developmental environments – a circumstance that may be altered through early intervention programmes.

Consequently, a reasonable expectation regarding the benefits of intervention beginning as early as possible is to prevent or substantially minimize this continuing decline in intellectual development. Indeed, this is precisely what occurs. Evidence from longitudinal studies from Australia (Berry *et al.* 1984), Israel (Sharav and Shlomo 1986), the United States (Schnell 1984) and Wales (Woods *et al.* 1984) indicates that comprehensive early intervention programmes can substantially prevent this decline in intellectual development from occurring for children with DS. Despite sometimes extensive differences in programme content and related factors, and the existence of legitimate methodological concerns (Gibson and Fields 1984; Guralnick and Bricker 1987), effect sizes of approximately one-half to three-quarters of a standard deviation are obtained in these studies of children with DS. Moreover, compatibility with findings from other risk and disability groups provides additional indirect support for the effectiveness of early intervention (Guralnick 1991).

## 10.3 Components of Early Intervention Programmes

The heterogeneity of intervention approaches and strategies found in programmes for children with DS, coupled with the fact that analyses of individual programme components were rarely conducted, did not permit an identification of those features of early intervention programmes that were responsible for the positive outcomes. Nevertheless, as these early intervention programmes evolved, a number of common features became established, thereby providing some insight into those components that, taken together, are likely to have promoted development. Specifically, systematic and usually highly structured and individualized programmes following curricula based on developmental milestones were common. Educational and developmental programmes were carried out at home and in specialized centres, and individual therapies were provided, especially physical therapy. Anticipatory guidance from professionals provided a wealth of information on education and health issues and strong parent-to-parent networks provided emotional, instrumental, and other forms of support (Guralnick and Bricker 1987). Information obtained from descriptive studies of the development of children with DS as well as research on parent-child interaction patterns appropriately formed the basis for specific intervention recommendations to foster more supportive, contingent, and sensitive transactions occurring between parents and children. Advice and strategies to help parents identify the often difficult-to-read cues of their child, to adapt to frequently hard-to-obtain eye contact, to adjust to episodes of vocal clashing during early parent-child 'conversational' interactions, to enhance environmental stimulation in an effort to almost drive development and encourage self-action, and to accommodate to the child's arousal and information-processing capacities constituted key elements of these programmes (Guralnick and Bricker 1987; Spiker 1990). As Spiker (1990) noted, much of the emphasis was on cognitive and language development, although other developmental areas have certainly been of interest. Moreover, parents were often enlisted as adjuncts in this intervention process, carrying out prescribed exercises and activities. Taken together, this array of components appeared capable of preventing continuing declines in overall development for children with DS in comparison with circumstances in which virtually no coordinated services existed, support and information were minimal, and community expectations were typically low.

## 10.4 Future Directions

Having said this, the issue that immediately arises is whether this is all that we can accomplish. Is it, in fact, possible to enhance further the effectiveness of early intervention programmes for children and families? If so, what directions should be pursued, and do we have any basis for optimism?

Perhaps what is needed is not a change in the content or components of early intervention programmes, but rather simply an increase in the intensity of what currently exists. After all, the formal aspects of early intervention programmes for children with DS are not very demanding, even during the preschool years (Guralnick and Bricker 1987; Shonkoff *et al.* 1992). Moreover, programme intensity seems to be an important dimension for children with other disabilities. Young children with autism appear to be remarkably responsive to extraordinarily intensive interventions, producing gains that are sustained over substantial periods of time (Lovaas 1987; McEachin *et al.* 1993). A replication of this highly intensive early intervention programme is now in progress for children with mild to moderate developmental delays with positive, though preliminary, findings being reported (Smith and Lovaas 1993). Unfortunately, children with DS were excluded in this investigation. Similarly, intensity appears to be an important factor contributing to the effectiveness of preventive intervention programmes for children at-risk due to prematurity and low birthweight (Ramey *et al.* 1992). Interestingly, for disadvantaged children, intensity in the form of programmes of longer duration (i.e., extending beyond the preschool years) has produced positive effects on assessed intellectual development and academic achievement that remain even after the intervention has been discontinued (Campbell and Ramey 1994; Reynolds 1994). The durability of gains from early intervention has been a major concern for children with DS (Gibson and Harris 1988), thereby warranting consideration of more intensive and/or extended interventions.

Alternatively, it may be advisable to reorganize content areas and instructional strategies in light of recent developmental research. For example, a stronger emphasis on memory, consolidation of skills, or motivational aspects of children with DS are potentially important directions (Wishart 1993). Moreover, it may be especially constructive to refocus the content of early intervention programmes entirely and to give priority to areas of development other than cognition or language. As argued elsewhere (Guralnick 1990a), a focus on promoting children's social competence, especially competence with peers, may be of particular value. This long-neglected area may offer special promise for children with DS, and is discussed below.

## 10.5 Peer-Related Social Competence

Developing peer relations and establishing friendships is a critical developmental task that is a challenge to all young children at some level during the preschool years. Parents of children with and without disabilities highly value and are concerned about this aspect of their child's development (Guralnick *et al.* 1995; Quirk *et al.* 1984). Successfully developing relationships with peers and establishing friendships has important developmental implications as well, with benefits associated with cognitive, communicative, and general prosocial development, as well as an emerging sense of self (Bates 1975; Garvey 1986; Hartup 1983; Howes 1988; Rubin and Lollis 1988). The importance of peer-related social competence as a determinant of social integration and social acceptance in classroom and community settings, as well as its importance to later life adjustment, has also been well established (Guralnick 1992).

In view of the developmental significance of peer-related social competence, it is discouraging to note the unusual difficulties experienced by young children with developmental disabilities in this domain. The limited social contacts and friendships reported for children with DS (Sloper *et al.* 1990) parallel reports for diverse groups of children with disabilities (Lewis *et al.* 1988). Moreover, a substantial body of research confirms that these difficulties are likely to be a consequence of problems associated with an unusual pattern of social interaction deficits. Indeed, particularly for children with general (cognitive) delays, including those with DS, problems in peer-related social competence extend well beyond those which would be expected based simply on a child's developmental level (Guralnick and Groom 1985, 1987, 1988).

## 10.6 Family Processes

Given the developmental significance and magnitude of the problem, can early intervention programmes foster the peer-related social competence of young children with DS? What information is available that might suggest particular directions? One highly active contemporary area of research focuses on the linkage between caregiver–child relationships and children's subsequent social competence, particularly peer-related social competence. This linkage between family processes and social competence has been well established (Guralnick and Neville, in press, for a review), with patterns holding for early caregiver-child relationships, typically evaluated in terms of the security of attachment relationships, as well as for subsequent interactions that emerge during the late toddler and preschool years. Indeed, recent research related to both attachment and later parent-child interactions for children with DS and their families suggests intervention directions that may well benefit children's peer-related social competence.

### 10.6.1 Attachment relationships

The quality of attachment formed between children and parents has yielded consistent associations with children's peer-related social competence in general (Cohn 1990; La Freniere and Sroufe 1985; Pastor 1981), as well as friendships (Elicker *et al.* 1992; Grossman and Grossman 1991). Moreover, a number of explanations for the effects of the secure attachment–social competence association have been put forward, including generalization of an 'internal working model' to other relationships, formation of a generalized positive social orientation, and availability of a secure base from which children can confidently explore both the physical and social world. The development of reciprocity patterns and enhancement of self-efficacy have also been implicated (see detailed discussion in Guralnick and Neville, in press).

Early research by Cicchetti and Serafica (1981) provided evidence that, in accordance with developmental levels, attachment relationships were organized in a similar manner for children with and without DS. Yet recent research has revealed that rather disturbing differences may well exist with regard to the attachment-related behaviour of children with DS (Vaughn *et al.* 1994). In particular, during the separation/reunion episodes that are central to the attachment assessment protocol, a disproportionate number of children with DS fail to show expected levels of distress and rarely seek contact or proximity with their mothers. Social cues that most typically-developing children exhibit to elicit parental behaviours of comforting are far less evident. These rather dramatic differences are likely due to many factors, including dampened arousal mechanisms (Emde *et al.* 1978). It appears that, although the meaning of attachment and its measurement are problematic for children with DS, the patterns observed by Vaughn *et al.* (1994) nevertheless remain a challenge to the emergence of harmonious and synchronous early parent-child relationships.

In view of associations between the early caregiver-child interactions and later social competence, a more focused and substantial effort by early interventionists to foster early caregiver-child relationships may prove to be a fruitful direction for the future. Some promising approaches for high-risk populations are available (Lieberman *et al.* 1991; van den Boom 1994), but the problems unique to children with DS, particularly emotional expressiveness and readability, will require highly imaginative early intervention strategies.

### 10.6.2 Parent-child interactions

The quality of parent-child interactions occurring during the late toddler and preschool period is also predictive of the quality of children's peer-related social competence (Guralnick 1986; Guralnick and Neville, in press). The parent-child dyad provides the context for learning and practising interpersonal skills that are relevant to the peer context (Martinez 1987). In fact, children are more likely to influence successfully the behaviour of their mothers in comparison to the behaviour of peers (Kochanska 1992), thereby having an opportunity to develop important social skills in the parent context related to social tasks such as conflict resolution or maintaining social exchanges. The parents' role in eliciting affective responses from their child during parent–child play has also been associated with children's peer-related social competence (see Parke *et al.*, 1992). Apparently, regulating one's emotions in the context of social play, indicating an ability to encode and decode emotions, serves an important role in developing social competence. As might be expected, contrasting parental styles such as those dominated by controlling or intrusive relationships are associated with lower levels of peer-related social competence for their children (Putallaz 1987).

Accordingly, the frequently observed tendency of many parents of young children with disabilities, including parents of children with DS, to adopt more controlling and directive styles while interacting with their children poses a potential concern for children's peer-related social competence (Mahoney *et al.* 1990). Admittedly, the nature and implications of this directive pattern are controversial (Marfo 1990). For example, individual differences are extensive, directive patterns may actually reflect an appropriate adjustment to less interactive children in many instances, and directive patterns must be understood in a broader context of parent–child relationships that include dimensions of warmth, sensitivity, and responsivity (Berger 1990; Crawley and Spiker 1983; Landry *et al.* 1994). However this is resolved, there nevertheless appears to be a substantial subset of parents of children with DS who exhibit a performance-oriented pattern of parent–child interactions, frequently seeking to elicit from their child some behaviour at as high a level of competence as possible (Mahoney *et al.* 1992). The resulting directive and controlling relationship may well create a pattern in which reciprocity and playfulness are relegated to minor roles, and fail to permit a child to develop an interaction pattern based on his or her own interests. These circumstances are inconsistent with fostering a child's ability to relate with peers (see Guralnick and Neville, in press).

Once again, it is this type of information that provides direction for future intervention strategies for families of children with DS during the early years. In this case, the challenge is first to develop tools sensitive enough to identify families exhibiting interaction patterns that may be counterproductive, and then to design appropriate interventions that do not themselves intrude or damage the core parent–child relationship. Interventions in this area will constitute a demanding test for the parent-professional partnership.

## 10.7 Improving Children's Peer-Related Social Competence: Child Focus

Successful interventions guided by recent developmental research to foster attachment and parent–child interactions may well prove beneficial for children's peer-related social competence, at least to some extent. Moreover, thoughtful efforts to expand the peer social network of a child with DS and interventions that support social exchanges with peers in high quality inclusive settings can also be of value (Buysse and Bailey 1993; Guralnick 1990b), as experience with peers is so critical for furthering the development of peer-related social competence. Yet, I would suggest that even if interventions based on family processes and the expansion of a child's social network are successful, substantial difficulties beyond those expected based on the child's developmental level (or language level) will remain. Recent advances in theory and research have led to a more in-depth understanding of cognitive and emotional regulation processes governing young children's peer-related social competence, and these are relevant to children with and without disabilities. Unfortunately, many of these underlying processes are likely to pose special difficulties for children with DS, suggesting that improvements in peer-related social competence will require highly sophisticated efforts that are child focused and consider these processes directly.

Figure 10.1 captures the key elements of a model I have developed over the last few years to guide the development of an assessment and intervention programme in the area of peer-related social competence (Guralnick 1992). Although it is beyond the scope of this chapter to provide an in-depth discussion, a consideration of its elements provides a sense for the issues involved (Dodge 1991; Dodge *et al.* 1986; Guralnick 1992, 1993, 1994).

First, as suggested by the bracketed area on the right of Figure 10.1, peer-related social competence is best thought of as being composed of a series of social tasks. In fact, three social tasks have been identified in the literature as being central to our understanding of peer-related social competence. These tasks are:

1. Gaining entry into a peer group;
2. Resolving conflicts;
3. Maintaining play with peers.

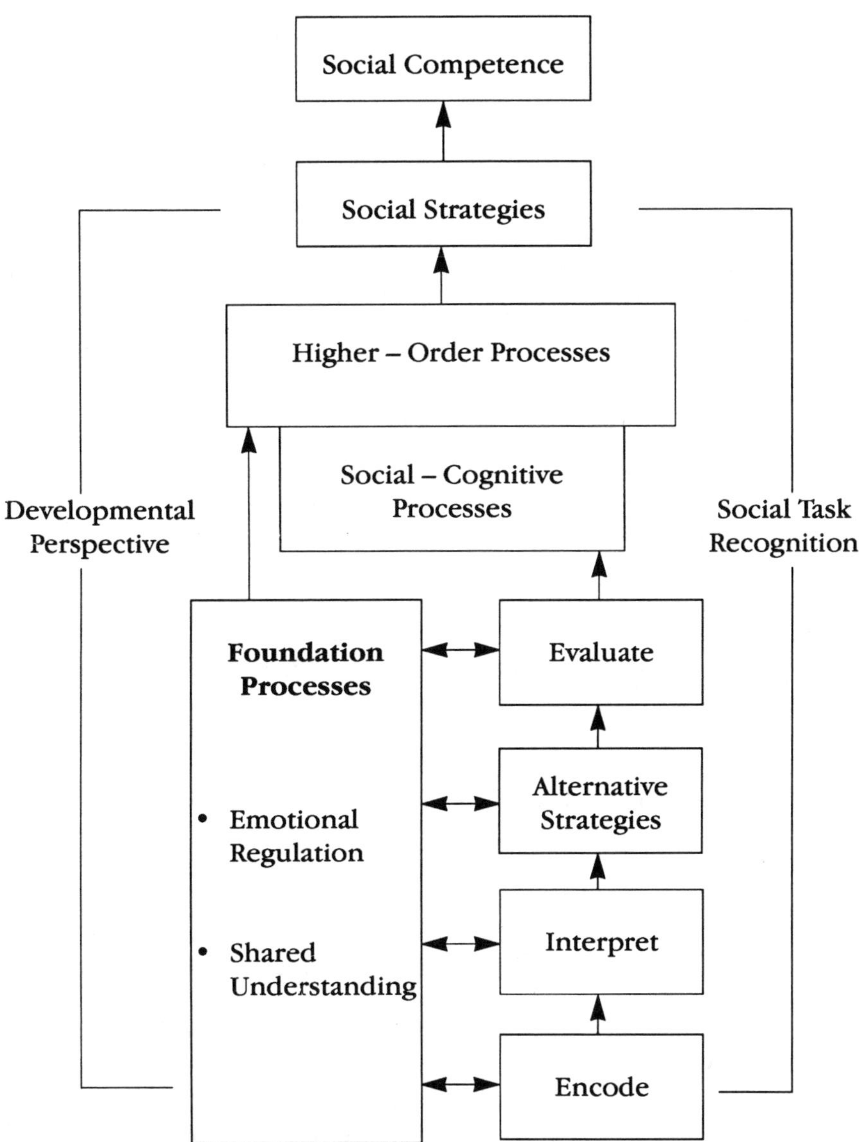


*Figure 10.1* A process model of peer-related social competence. From: Assessment of Peer Relations, MJ Guralnick 1991, Seattle WA: University of Washington, Center on Human Development and Disability. Reprinted by permission.

Competence is typically evaluated in the context of one or more of these social tasks in terms of the effectiveness and appropriateness of the social strategies that are employed. These social strategies, in turn, depend upon the operation of four interrelated processes. The first two processes are referred to as foundation processes. One involves the pattern employed by a child to regulate his or her emotions during a social task. The unusual problems experienced by children with DS, ranging from often reported lower arousal to difficulties settling once an emotional event is triggered (see Cicchetti, Ganiban *et al.* 1991), are likely to be of special concern.

The other foundation process is referred to as shared understanding. Knowledge of sequences of behaviours (i.e., scripts) associated with everyday events (e.g., cooking) form the substance of dramatic play sequences. Moreover, mutually agreed upon and understood social rules (e.g., turn-taking, possession) are relevant, and together constitute the basis for connectedness essential for socially competent interactions with peers (Nelson 1986). For children with DS, memory and self-organizing difficulties as well as problems integrating social and non-social activities required by scripts pose challenges to the development of a well-developed, shared understanding (Beeghly *et al.* 1989; Gibson 1992; Kopp 1990; Krakow and Kopp 1983; Mundy *et al.* 1988).

The last two processes (see Figure 10.1) emphasize the information-processing components of the model. Social-cognitive processes are composed of elements related to how children encode information, interpret it, produce alternative strategies, and evaluate those strategies in terms of the context. Similarly, a higher order process proposed as an integrator of this information requires that children recognize the social task they are engaged in, sustain attention, and monitor outcomes. Available neuropsychological models of social competence are consistent with this approach (Pennington and Welsh 1995).

It is precisely those deficits in information-processing (Lincoln *et al.* 1985), verbal coding and decoding (Gibson 1992), failures to produce alternative types of strategies in related tasks (Kopp *et al.* 1983), and to recognize emotional expressions (Knieps *et al.* 1994) that again create special problems for children with DS. Moreover, Wishart (1993) states: 'From a very early age, it would appear that the DS [Down's syndrome] children are avoiding opportunities for learning new skills, making poor use of skills that are acquired, and failing to consolidate skills into their repertoires' (p. 400). These new as well as longstanding motivational and learning style issues which Wishart has now put into perspective for children with DS are even apparent in early exploratory object play (Ruskin, *et al.* 1994a,b). Clearly, difficulties observed during cognitive tasks are likely to adversely influence social tasks that rely on social-cognitive processes.

Having now developed a better understanding of the processes likely to affect children's peer-related social competence, the critical question revolves around what approaches can be taken to intervene during the preschool years. At the present time, an intervention approach that focuses on techniques that adapt to problematic processes and provide structured experiences to enhance the peer-related social competence of young children with disabilities is being evaluated. Vignettes to foster script development for dramatic or even physical play sequences as well as for social task recognition have been developed. For children with DS, techniques involving social imitation, providing predictable and often repetitive sequences with variations in context, and arranging involvement with peers in small group settings are only some of the strategies being employed.

## 10.8 Conclusions

Considerable progress has been achieved in the field of early intervention for children with DS, particularly in terms of reducing the continuing decline in intellectual development over the first few years of life. However, we are now at a critical point, seeking to determine what more can be accomplished. Intervention research with other disability or risk populations suggests the possibility that increasing the intensity of interventions can produce further benefits, particularly enhancing the durability of effects. It is uncertain as to whether that also will be the case for children with DS. Alternatively, an emphasis on promoting children's peer-related social competence, an area of special concern, through a combination of parent- and child-focused strategies may prove to be fruitful. Programmes developed in response to recent developmental information on parent–child relationships, children's learning styles, as well as cognitive and emotional processes associated with children with DS constitute important directions for early intervention research and practice.

## References

Bates E (1975) Peer relations and the acquisition of language. In M Lewis and L A Rosenblum (Eds) The origins of behavior: Vol.4. Friendship and peer relations, pp. 259–92. New York: John Wiley and Sons.

Beeghly M, Weiss-Perry B and Cicchetti, D (1989) Structural and affective dimensions of play development on young children with Down syndrome. International Journal of Behavioral Development 12: 257–77.

Bendersky M and Lewis M (1994) Environmental risk, biological risk, and developmental outcome. Developmental Psychology 30: 484–94.

Berger J (1990) Interactions between parents and their infants with Down syndrome. In D Cicchetti and M Beeghly (Eds) Children with Down syndrome: A developmental perspective, pp.101–46. Cambridge: Cambridge University Press.

Berry P, Gunn VP and Andrews R J (1984) Development of Down's syndrome children from birth to five years. In JM Berg (Ed) Perspectives and progress in mental retardation: Vol. 1. Social, psychological, and educational aspects, pp.167–77. Baltimore: University Park Press.

Brooks-Gunn J, Klebanov PK, Liaw F and Spiker D (1993) Enhancing the development of low-birthweight, premature infants: changes in cognition and behavior over the first three years. Child Development 64: 736–53.

Buysse V and Bailey DB Jr (1993) Behavioral and developmental outcomes in young children with disabilities in integrated and segregated settings: A review of comparative studies. The Journal of Special Education, 26: 434-61.

Campbell FA and Ramey CT (1994) Effects of early intervention on intellectual and academic achievement: A follow-up study of children from low-income families. Child Development 65: 684–98.

Carr J (1970) Mental and motor development in young mongol children. Journal of Mental Deficiency Research 14: 205.

Cicchetti D, Ganiban G and Barnett D (1991) Contributions from the study of high-risk populations to understanding the development of emotion regulation. In J Garber and KA Dodge (Eds) The development of emotion regulation and dysregulation, pp.15–48. New York: Cambridge University Press.

Cicchetti D and Serafica FC (1981) Interplay among behavioral systems: Illustrations from the study of attachment, affiliation, and wariness in young children with Down's syndrome. Developmental Psychology 17: 36–49.

Cohn DA (1990) Child–mother attachment of six-year-olds and social competence at school. Child Development 61: 152–62.

Connolly JA (1978) Intelligence levels of Down's syndrome children. American Journal of Mental Deficiency 83: 193–6.

Crawley SB and Spiker D (1983) Mother–child interactions involving two-year-olds with Down syndrome: A look at individual differences. Child Development 54: 1312–23.

Dodge KA (1991) Emotion and social information processing. In J Garber and KA Dodge (Eds) The development of emotion regulation and dysregulation, pp.159–81. New York: Cambridge University Press.

Dodge KA, Pettit GS, McClaskey CL and Brown MM (1986) Social competence in children. Monographs of the Society for Research in Child Development 51: (2, Serial No. 213).

Dunst CJ, Trivette CM and Cross AH (1986) Mediating influences of social support: Personal, family, and child outcomes. American Journal of Mental Deficiency 90: 403–17.

Elicker J, Englund M and Sroufe LA (1992) Predicting peer competence and peer relationships in childhood from early parent-child relationships. In RD Parke and GW Ladd (Eds) Family-peer relationships: Modes of linkage, pp.77–106. Hillsdale NJ: Erlbaum.

Emde RN, Katz EL and Thorpe JK (1978) Emotional expression in infancy: II. Early deviations in Down's syndrome. In M Lewis and LA Rosenblum (Eds) The development of affect, pp.351–60. New York: Plenum.

Garvey C (1986) Peer relations and the growth of communication. In EC Mueller and CR Cooper (Eds) Process and outcome in peer relationships, pp.329–45. Orlando FL: Academic Press.

Gibson D (1992) Down syndrome and cognitive enhancement: Not like the others. In K Marfo (Ed) Early intervention in transition: Current perspectives on programs for handicapped children, pp.61–90. New York: Praeger.

Gibson D and Fields DL (1984) Early infant stimulation programs for children with Down syndrome: A review of effectiveness. In M Wolraich and DK Routh (Eds) Advances in developmental and behavioral pediatrics 5: pp 331–71. Greenwich, CT: JAI Press.

Gibson D and Harris A (1988) Aggregated early intervention effects for Down's syndrome persons: patterning and longevity of benefits. Journal of Mental Deficiency Research 32: 1-17.

Grossman KE and Grossman K (1991) Attachment quality as an organizer of emotional and behavioral responses. In C Parkes, J Stevenson-Hinde and P Marris (Eds) Attachment across the life cycle, pp.93–114. New York: Routledge.

Guralnick MJ (1986) The peer relations of young handicapped and nonhandicapped children. In PS Strain, MJ Guralnick and HM Walker (Eds) Children's social behavior: Development, assessment, and modification, pp.93–140. New York: Academic Press.

Guralnick MJ (1990a) Social competence and early intervention. Journal of Early Intervention 14: 3–14.

Guralnick MJ (1990b) Major accomplishments and future directions in early childhood mainstreaming. Topics in Early Childhood Special Education 10: 1–17.

Guralnick MJ (1991) The next decade of research on the effectiveness of early intervention. Exceptional Children 58: 174–83.

Guralnick MJ (1992) A hierarchical model for understanding children's peer-related social competence. In SL Odom, SR McConnell, and MA McEvoy (Eds) Social competence of young children with disabilities: Issues and strategies for intervention, pp.37–64. Baltimore: Brookes.

Guralnick MJ (1993) Developmentally appropriate practice in the assessment and intervention of children's peer relations. Topics in Early Childhood Special Education 13: 344–71.

Guralnick MJ (1994) Social competence with peers: Outcome and process in early childhood special education. In PL Safford (Ed) Yearbook in early childhood education: Early childhood special education Vol. 5: pp 45–71. New York: Teacher's College Press.

Guralnick MJ (Ed) (in press) The effectiveness of early intervention: Directions for second generation research. Baltimore: Brookes.

Guralnick MJ and Bricker D (1987) The effectiveness of early intervention for children with cognitive and general developmental delays. In MJ Guralnick and FC Bennett (Eds) The effectiveness of early intervention for at-risk and handicapped children, pp.115–73. New York: Academic Press.

Guralnick MJ, Connor R and Hammond M (1995) Parent perspectives of peer relations and friendships in integrated and specialized programs. American Journal on Mental Retardation 99: 457–76.

Guralnick MJ and Groom JM (1985) Correlates of peer-related social competence of developmentally delayed preschool children. American Journal of Mental Deficiency 90: 140–50.

Guralnick MJ and Groom JM (1987) The peer relations of mildly delayed and nonhandicapped preschool children in mainstreamed playgroups. Child Development 58: 1556–72.

Guralnick MJ and Groom JM (1988) Friendships of preschool children in mainstreamed playgroups. Developmental Psychology 24: 595–604.

Guralnick MJ and Neville B (in press) Designing early intervention programs to promote children's social competence. In MJ Guralnick (Ed) The effectiveness of early intervention. Baltimore: Brookes.

Hartup WW (1983) Peer relations. In EM Hetherington (Ed) PH Mussen (Series Ed) Handbook of child psychology: Vol. 4. Socialization, personality, and social development, pp.103–96. New York: Wiley.

Howes C (1988) Peer interaction of young children. Monographs of the Society for Research in Child Development 53: (1, Serial No. 217).

Knieps LJ, Walden TA and Baxter A (1994) Affective expressions of toddlers with and without Down syndrome in a social referencing context. American Journal on Mental Retardation 99: 301–12.

Kochanska G (1992) Children's interpersonal influence with mothers and peers. Developmental Psychology 28: 491–9.

Kopp CB (1990) The growth of self-monitoring among young children with Down syndrome. In D Cicchetti and M Beeghly (Eds) Children with Down syndrome: A developmental perspective, pp.231–51. New York: Cambridge University Press.

Kopp CB, Krakow JB and Johnson KL (1983) Strategy production by young Down syndrome children. American Journal of Mental Deficiency 88: 164–9.

Krakow JB and Kopp CB (1983) The effects of developmental delay on sustained attention in young children. Child Development 54: 1143-55.

La Freniere PJ and Sroufe LA (1985) Profiles of peer competence in the preschool: Interrelations between measures, influence of social ecology, and relation to attachment history. Developmental Psychology 21: 56–69.

Landry SH, Garner PW, Pirie D and Swank PR (1994) Effects of social context and mothers' requesting strategies on Down's syndrome children's social responsiveness. Developmental Psychology 30: 293–302.

Lewis M, Feiring C and Brooks-Gunn J (1988) Young children's social networks as a function of age and dysfunction. Infant Mental Health Journal 9: 142–57.

Liaw F-R and Brooks-Gunn J (1993) Patterns of low-birth-weight children's cognitive development. Developmental Psychology 29: 1024–35.

Lieberman AF, Weston DR and Pawl JH (1991) Preventive intervention and outcome with anxiously attached dyads. Child Development 62: 199–209.

Lincoln AJ, Courchesne E, Kilman BA and Galambos R (1985) Neuropsychological correlates of information-processing by children with Down syndrome. American Journal of Mental Deficiency 89: 403–14.

Lovaas OI (1987) Behavioral treatment and normal educational and intellectual functioning in young autistic children. Journal of Consulting and Clinical Psychology 55: 3–9.

Mahoney GJ, Fors S and Wood S (1990) Maternal directive behavior revisited. American Journal on Mental Retardation 94: 398–406.

Mahoney G, Robinson C and Powell A (1992) Focusing on parent-child interaction: The bridge to developmentally appropriate practices. Topics in Early Childhood Special Education 12: 105–20.

Marfo K (1990) Maternal directiveness in interactions with mentally handicapped children: An analytical commentary. Journal of Child Psychology and Psychiatry 31: 531–49.

Martinez MA (1987) Dialogues among children and between children and their mothers. Child Development 58: 1035–43.

McEachin JJ, Smith T and Lovaas OI (1993) Long-term outcome for children with autism who received early intensive behavioral treatment. American Journal on Mental Retardation 97: 359–72.

Melyn MA and White DT (1973) Mental and developmental milestones of noninstitutionalized Down's syndrome children. Pediatrics 52: 542–5.

Morgan SB (1979) Development and distribution of intellectual and adaptive skills in Down syndrome children: Implications for early intervention. Mental Retardation 17: 247–9.

Mundy P, Sigman M, Kasari C and Yirmiya N (1988) Nonverbal communication skills in Down syndrome children. Child Development 59: 235–49.

Nelson K (Ed) (1986) Event knowledge: Structure and function in development. Hillsdale NJ: Erlbaum.

Neser PSJ, Molteno CD and Knight GJ (1989) Evaluation of preschool children with

Down's syndrome in Cape Town using the Griffiths Scale of Mental Development. Child: Care, Health and Development 15: 217–25.

Palmer FB, Shapiro BK, Wachtel RC, Allen MC, Hiller JE, Harryman SE, Mosher BS, Meinert CL and Capute AJ (1988) The effects of physical therapy on cerebral palsy. New England Journal of Medicine 318: 803–8.

Parke RD, Cassidy J, Burks VM, Carson JL and Boyum L (1992) Familial contributions to peer competence among young children: The role of interactive and affective processes. In RD Parke and GW Ladd (Eds) Family-peer relationships: Modes of linkage, pp.107–34. Hillsdale NJ: Erlbaum.

Pastor DL (1981) The quality of mother-infant attachment and its relationship to toddlers' initial sociability with peers. Developmental Psychology 17: 326–35.

Pennington BF and Welsh M (1995) Neuropsychology and developmental psychopathology. In D Cicchetti and D Cohen (Eds) Handbook of developmental psychopathology, pp.254–90. New York: Cambridge University Press.

Putallaz M (1987) Maternal behavior and children's sociometric status. Child Development 58: 324–40.

Quirk M, Sexton M, Ciottone R, Minami H and Wapner S (1984) Values held by mothers for handicapped and nonhandicapped preschoolers. Merrill-Palmer Quarterly 30: 403–18.

Ramey CT, Bryant DM, Wasik BH, Sparling JJ, Fendt KH and La Vange LM (1992) Infant health and development program for low birth weight, premature infants: Program elements, family participation, and child intelligence. Pediatrics 89: 454–65.

Rauh VA, Achenbach TM, Nurcombe B, Howell CT and Teti DM (1988) Minimizing adverse effects of low birthweight: Four-year results of an early intervention program. Child Development 59: 544–53.

Reynolds AJ (1994) Effects of a preschool plus follow-on intervention for children at risk. Developmental Psychology 30: 787–804.

Rubin KH and Lollis SP (1988) Origins and consequences of social withdrawal. In J Belsky and T Nezworski (Eds) Clinical implications of attachment, pp.219–52. Hillsdale NJ: Erlbaum.

Ruskin EM, Kasari C, Mundy P and Sigman M (1994a) Attention to people and toys during social and object mastery in children with Down syndrome. American Journal on Mental Retardation 99: 103–11.

Ruskin EM, Mundy P, Kasari C and Sigman M (1994b) Object mastery motivation of children with Down syndrome. American Journal on Mental Retardation 98: 499–509.

Schnell R (1984) Psychomotor development. In S Peuschel (Ed) The young child with Down syndrome, pp.207–26. New York: Human Sciences.

Sharav T and Shlomo L (1986) Stimulation of infants with Down syndrome: Long-term effects. Mental Retardation 24: 81–6.

Shonkoff JP, Hauser-Cram P, Krauss MW and Upshur CC (1992) Development of infants with disabilities and their families. Monographs of the Society for Research in Child Development 57: (6, Serial No. 230).

Sloper P, Turner S, Knussen C and Cunningham C (1990) Social life of school children with Down's syndrome. Child: Care, Health and Development 16: 235–51.

Smith T and Lovaas OI (1993) Intensive behavioral treatment of young children with mild to moderate mental retardation. Unpublished Interim Report on Office of Education Grant H133G80103, University of California, Los Angeles.

Spiker D (1990) Early intervention from a developmental perspective. In D Cicchetti and M Beeghly (Eds) Children with Down syndrome: A developmental perspective, pp.424–48. New York: Cambridge University Press.

van den Boom DC (1994) The influence of temperament and mothering on attachment and exploration: An experimental manipulation of sensitive responsiveness among lower-class mothers and irritable infants. Child Development 65: 1457–77.

Vaughn BE, Goldberg S, Atkinson L, Marcovitch S, MacGregor D and Seifer R (1994) Quality of toddler-mother attachment in children with Down syndrome: Limits to interpretation of strange situation behavior. Child Development 65: 95–108.

Wishart JG (1993) The development of learning difficulties in children with Down's syndrome. Journal of Intellectual Disability Research 37: 389–403.

Woods PA, Corney MJ and Pryce GJ (1984) Developmental progress of preschool Down's syndrome children receiving a home-advisory service: An interim report. Child: Care, Health and Development 10: 287–99.

# Part Five: Personality and Development

# 11 Socio-affective Development in Infants with Down's Syndrome

ISIDORO CANDEL GIL, JOSÉ ANTONIO CARRANZA CARNICERO, JULIO PÉREZ LÓPEZ

## 11.1 Introduction

Studies on the socio-affective development of Down's syndrome (DS) infants confirm the presence of evolutional patterns similar to non-delayed infants. They also emphasise several qualitative differences. From an organizational perspective, cognitive and affective developments appear to be two inseparable aspects of the same developmental process (Cicchetti and Sroufe 1978). As we shall see, the qualitative differences observed with regard to non-delayed children cannot be explained by cognitive factors only. These differences mark a developmental rate and specific behavioural characteristics which determine the degree of interaction of the DS infant with his or her physical and social environment.

A brief look at the study of development in DS infants reveals that these infants have the same organization of affective and cognitive skills and follow the same developmental patterns as non-delayed infants. This is the case in such different areas as discrimination and expression of emotions (Cicchetti and Sroufe 1976, 1978; Sorce and Emde 1982; Berger and Cunningham 1986; Loeches 1988); reaction to separation from the mother and towards a stranger (Berry *et al.* 1980; Cicchetti and Serafica 1981); self-cognition (Cicchetti and Sroufe 1978); behaviour which the infants develop during play activities (Motti *et al.* 1983; Beeghly *et al.* 1989) and the capacity for generalizing experiences (MacTurk *et al.* 1985).

However, important qualitative differences can also be observed. Primarily, there is a developmental delay in DS compared with non-delayed infants in all of the aforementioned areas. In the case of positive emotion, it is observed that affective behaviour in DS infants is less intense. They tend to smile rather than laugh, this being more common with the more hypotonic infants. The same can be said for negative emotions, where the infants with a higher level of development show more intense emotional reactions (fear, shouting) than the more hypotonic infants with lower development levels. With regard to social-interaction behaviour, DS infants take fewer initiatives and do not tend to take the lead in social interaction. They also respond less to their mothers and produce fewer socio-communicative behaviours, such as sharing or giving. It therefore seems that DS infants are not as efficient as non-delayed infants in the use of their behavioural capacities in order to relate to the social environment and draw information from it.

Many of these qualitative differences in DS infants cannot be explained by cognitive factors alone. Their origin seems to be in the activity of the central and peripheral transmission systems, which play an important role in the regulation of reactivity to stimulation. In an interesting review, Ganiban *et al.* (1990) discuss the neurological limitations that can explain many of the qualitative differences observed throughout the development process of DS infants:

- In the central nervous system (CNS) of people with DS there is a decrease both in the number of cells and cholinergic levels. It is possible that the decrease in acetylcholine in the CNS of people with DS reflects a difference in their general capacity of responding to the environment.
- In people with DS there is also a decrease in serotonin levels, which implies that these people may find it difficult to regulate sleep–awake cycles.
- In addition, there seems to be a decrease in noradrenaline production in individuals with DS, which can imply a decrease in sensitivity to novelty in their environment, as well as a general decrease in the activation of the sympathetic nervous system.
- The genetic disturbance characteristic of DS can also affect the liberation of neurotransmitters in the blood stream via the endocrine systems. These possible differences in the activity of the neurotransmitter systems as well as in neuroanatomical structures suggest the presence of fundamental constitutional differences in the reactivity of individuals with DS.

## 11.2 Approximation to Temperament Study

In the area of socio-affective development, the study of temperament is becoming increasingly more important. Indeed, the existence of individual differences in the way in which infants relate to their surroundings as well as the nature and affective tone of their interaction has provided new starting points for the interpretation of the contributions of the infants themselves to their social and emotional development.

Despite the growing interest in recent years in the study of temperament in infancy, there still does not exist a clear definition which encompasses the different interpretations of the substance and meaning of temperament. Thomas and Chess (1977) emphasize the stylistic character of temperament, i.e., not what the person does but how he or she does it. Buss and Plomin (1984) have a similar view. Accordingly, temperament refers to the stylistic aspects of behaviour, i.e.; how the response is carried out (fast or slow, smooth or intense, etc.). However, they also point out that temperamental characteristics must be inherited and show up from early age.

Despite this wide range of interpretations about temperament, we are able to point out some common characterisitics:

- Temperamental dimensions reflect behavioural trends, not discrete behavioural actions;
- Temperament consists of basic dispositions inherent to the individual which have a biological/constitutional base, although the authors' opinions differ in the degree to which these characteristics are assumed to be genetic in their source, and also in the degree to which they are modifiable. The main attributes of temperament are present from an early stage in life. As development takes place, the expression of temperament is increasingly influenced by experience and context;
- There appears to be a continuity in temperament throughout life when compared with other aspects of behaviour;
- Among the many temperamental characteristics proposed by the various theories on temperament, activity, emotionality and sociability play some part in the majority of temperament dimensions.

In any case, as Lerner (1993) suggests, temperament characteristics have been thought of as valid dimensions of individuality according to the effects of the infant on others, the transactional relationships of the infant with his social context, and the means by which the infant can promote his own development.

## 11.3 Temperament in Down's Syndrome Infants

As we have already seen, possible differences in the activity of neurotransmitter systems and neuroanatomic structures suggest the presence of fundamental constitutional differences in the reactivity of people with DS. Differences in the basic functioning of the central and peripheral nervous systems can be seen to influence underlying emotionality in the form of a diminished sensitivity towards what is new, and a smaller capacity of response to the environment. It is not surprising that DS infants initially respond with less intensity to external events and that their diminished sensitivity towards what is new makes them seem less sensitive to change and more stubborn or persistent in their behaviour (Flórez 1995).

During the first years of life, changes in reactivity are expected as the central and parasympathetic nervous systems mature. The growth, later development and differentiation of these systems lay the foundations of the ability for each system to voluntarily regulate arousal capacity and emotionality. Many studies have indicated that there are anomalies in the growth and elaboration of the nervous system during the postnatal period in DS (Kemper 1988; Wisniewski 1990). The brains of individuals with DS mature with less speed and extension (Flórez 1995). These problems in neurological maturation may have an influence on the development and appearance of temperamental characteristics. If the changes in temperament over time reflect the maturation of the CNS, it is to be expected that DS infants will not show the changes in temperament characteristics at the same times as non-delayed infants.

As Ganiban *et al.* (1990) correctly point out, studies of temperament in DS infants are justified for various reasons. One pragmatic motive is to obtain more information about the response characteristics in this population. Secondly, the early identifiability of the characteristics as well as the typical features of DS allow us to make inferences about the possible contribution of genetic and biological influences on behaviour. Thirdly, the discordance between intellectual development and chronological age (CA) allows us to examine the coherence of the organization of different capacities and their impact on the capacity for behavioural response.

The studies on temperament in DS infants started from the initial interpretation of the presence of certain temperamental stereotypes linked to distinct developmental stages. This led to a description of temperamental characteristics, emphasizing the homogeneity of the group more than the individual differences. Thus, individuals with DS have traditionally been considered stubborn but affectionate with an easy temperament. However, these stereotypes cannot be maintained when they are subjected to empirical investigation, as Gibson points out (1978). He concludes that the temperament of individuals with DS is not uniform, but that there is a wide range of temperament profiles, as occurs in other types of mental deficiency, and also in non-delayed individuals. Gibson attributes this temperamental variability in individuals with DS to genetic composition, response capacity, neurological maturation and intellectual status.

In short, a review of the different studies (Bridges and Cicchetti 1982; Rothbart and Hanson 1983; Gunn *et al.* 1983; Gunn and Berry 1985; Marcovitch *et al.* 1986; Goldberg and Marcovitch 1989; Vaughn *et al.* 1994) allows us to draw the following conclusions:

1. No significant differences between DS and non-delayed infants have been found in the temperament dimensions studied. However, it has been observed that DS infants between 0 and 3 years have a more difficult temperament than non-delayed infants of the same age.
2. With regards to temperament, DS infants appear to be similar to delayed infants of other etiologies. However, some differences in the variables of approach, activity and distractibility are observed.
3. There seems to be little stability in the temperament classifications in DS infants, as changes occur with age: DS infants between 0 and 3 years-old show a difficult temperament while those between 3 and 6 years-old seem to have an easier temperament. Infants considered as having an easy temperament are those who appear active, playful and docile in social interaction; on the other hand, infants with a difficult temperament show irregularity in their biological rates, avoidance of new situations, slow capacity of adaptation and a relatively negative mood.
4. There appears to exist a coincidence in some temperamental dimensions of DS infants as a group. For example, they tend to be more rhythmic, more uncontrollable, more adaptable and they score more highly in persistence. On the other hand, compared with control groups of non-delayed infants, they obtain lower scores in approach to objects, stimulation threshold, reaction to shock, vocal activity, intensity of response, and positive affect.
5. It is important to bear in mind that there is variability in the temperament profiles of DS infants. Therefore, as indicated by Goldber and Marcovitch (1989), a generalization or stereotype is of limited usefulness in understanding the infants' individually.

In short, there does not seem to be a single, homogeneous temperament profile in DS infants, but rather a wide variation among them. The stereotype of easy temperament and temperament homogeneity is not in any way confirmed. As a result, it is expected that individuals with DS show a wide range of temperament profiles and characteristics (Candel and Carranza 1993).

## 11.4 An Empirical Study

The study we shall present is part of an ongoing longitudinal investigation on temperament in DS infants. Sample selection has been based on mental age (MA) and not CA. We have already seen the importance of cognitive skills for understanding the responses of DS infants from an emotional and social viewpoint. In addition to the evaluation of temperamental characteristics, often carried out based on mothers' reports, we also propose an analysis of relevant laboratory tasks. Our study will also compare the response level of temperamental dimensions in DS infants with that of a sample of non-delayed infants. The particular objectives are as follows:

1. To study temperament components in successive periods of development in DS infants.
2. To evaluate the degree of stability /instability of individual differences in temperament components in DS infants.
3. To analyse the degree of homogeneity of temperamental characteristics in DS infants as a group and the differences with a group of non-delayed infants.

### 11.4.1 Subjects

The experimental subjects were twelve infants with Down's syndrome (DS) (5 girls and 7 boys) and their mothers. All DS infants were karyotyped as trisomy 21. They were evaluated as having 9 months of MA on the *Bayley Scales of Infant Development* (1977). Infants with severe medical or behavioural complications were excluded from the study. The control group was made up of sixty non-delayed infants (29 girls and 31 boys) MA-matched with the DS infants and their mothers. None of the infants experienced any prenatal nor postnatal complication. Direct measurements used the *Developmental Tasks and Rating Scales for the Laboratory Assessment of Infant Temperament* (Matheny and Wilson 1981). This test consists of a structured sequence of tasks linked to age, presented to the infant as challenges to cope with. The dimensions assessed were as follows:

*Emotional tone* i.e., the main emotional state exhibited during the rating period, ranging from extreme distress to animate laughter;
*Activity* i.e., body motion with or without locomotion, which could involve whole or partial movements;
*Social orientation to staff* i.e., the positive and negative aspects of social orientation of the infant in relation to others, with some emphasis on approach–avoidance behaviours;
*Attentiveness* i.e., the degree to which the infant was alert and maintained attention towards objects and events;
*Vocalizations* i.e., non-crying utterances or recognizable utterances embedded in crying; crying, per se, no matter how varied, did not qualify.

Indirect measurements were made through the *Rothbart's Infant Behaviour Questionnaire* (1981) was used. This questionnaire comprises 94 items. Parents are asked about their infant's behaviour in everyday situations such as care, play, sleeping. This questionnaire provides an infant's temperament profile based on six dimensions:

*Activity level* which implies the level of gross motor activity;

*Laughter and smiling* which have been identified as indicators of arousal under safe conditions;

*Fear*, reacting to sudden changes in stimulation and the latency in approaching new objects (physical or social);

*Distress faced with limitations*, a variable that reflects individual differences in infants' reactions to frustrating conditions;

*Duration of orientation* defined as vocalizations, looking at, and/or interacting with a single object when there has been no sudden change in stimulation; and, finally,

*Soothability* consisting of the infant's reduction to fussing, crying, or distress when soothing techniques are used by caretakers.

The first assessment for the infants with DS took place at 9 months MA. Three months later the infants were assessed again. Each of the assessments was videotaped for subsequent analysis by independent observers (interrater reliability was 0.98 using the Matheny and Wilson 1981 procedure). The IBQ questionnaires were filled in by the mothers on their visits to the laboratory.

The SYSTAT statistical package (version 5.0) was used for analysing the data. A Pearson product-moment correlation coefficient was computed between the scores in the stability of temperamental dimensions in laboratory tasks and the IBQ questionnaire. The results appears in Table 11.1 below.

Table 11.1 Pearson Product-moment Correlation Coefficient for laboratory tasks and IBQ questionnaires in infants with Down's syndrome and non-delayed infants at 9 and 12 months.

| *Laboratory Tasks* | 9 vs 12 months Down's syndrome | 9 vs 12 months non-delayed |
|---|---|---|
| Emotional tone | 0.59* | 0.52*** |
| Activity | 0.69* | 0.14 |
| Social orientation | 0.57 | 0.47* |
| Attentiveness | 0.42 | 0.46*** |
| *IBQ* | 9 vs. 12 months Down's syndrome | 9 vs. 12 months non-delayed |
| Level of activity | 0.64* | 0.47*** |
| Distress to limitations | 0.29 | 0.29* |
| Fear | 0.62* | 0.38** |
| Duration of orientation | 0.35 | 0.31* |
| Laughter/Smiling | 0.31 | 0.63*** |
| Soothability | 0.61* | – |

* = $p<0.05$
** = $p<0.01$
***= $p<0.001$

Table 11.2 Component loadings and percentage of total variance explained

| | *Infants with Down's Syndrome* | | | *Non-delayed Infants* | | |
|---|---|---|---|---|---|---|
| | 9 months | 12 months | 12 months | 9 months | 12 months | 12 months |
| | Factor I Tractability | Factor I Mood | Factor II Tractability | Factor I Tractability | Factor I Mood | Factor II Tractability |
| Emotional tone | 0.903 | 0.815 | 0.419 | 0.865 | 0.653 | 0.559 |
| Activity | 0.836 | 0.892 | 0.178 | 0.802 | 0.889 | –0.064 |
| Attentiveness | 0.836 | 0.279 | 0.788 | 0.831 | –0.026 | 0.914 |
| Social orientation | 0.826 | 0.012 | 0.865 | 0.830 | 0.028 | 0.888 |
| Vocalizations | 0.660 | 0.900 | –0.022 | 0.483 | 0.880 | 0.010 |
| % Variance explained | 66.63% | 46.95% | 31.54% | 60.11% | 39.84% | 38.83% |

A varimax-rotated principal components analysis (PCA) was computed on the scores in the laboratory tasks computed at each age. The aim of this analysis was to determine whether clusters of temperamental dimensions existed. The PCA of DS infants showed one factor at the age of 9 months, and two factors on the following assessment, three months later. These results were the same with non-delayed infants. The results are displayed in Table 11.2.

Finally, a comparison analysis was made between the means of the two samples of children. Results appear in Tables 11.3 and 11.4.

Table 11.3 Comparisons between means (X) in Down's syndrome and non-delayed infants at 9 and 12 months in laboratory tasks

9 months

| *Laboratory* | *X Down's* | *X Non-delayed* | *SD Down's* | *SD Non-delayed* | *Degree freedom* | *T* | *Probability* |
|---|---|---|---|---|---|---|---|
| Emotional tone | 5.425 | 5.791 | 0.627 | 0.562 | 68 | 2.075 | 0.042* |
| Activity | 4.642 | 4.670 | 0.813 | 0.694 | 68 | 0.125 | 0.901 |
| Social orientation | 5.957 | 5.963 | 0.428 | 0.300 | 68 | 0.062 | 0.951 |
| Attentiveness | 5.479 | 5.018 | 0.866 | 0.697 | 68 | –2.055 | 0.044* |
| Vocalizations | 3.092 | 2.321 | 1.710 | 0.746 | 68 | –2.539 | 0.013* |

12 months

| *Laboratory* | *X Down's* | *X Non-delayed* | *SD Down's* | *SD Non-delayed* | *Degree freedom* | *T* | *Probability* |
|---|---|---|---|---|---|---|---|
| Emotional tone | 5.361 | 5.969 | 0.516 | 0.598 | 67 | 3.274 | 0.002** |
| Activity | 4.579 | 5.325 | 1.011 | 0.859 | 67 | 2.650 | 0.010** |
| Social orientation | 6.020 | 6.199 | 0.331 | 0.370 | 67 | 1.547 | 0.127 |
| Attentiveness | 5.596 | 5.276 | 0.514 | 0.711 | 67 | –1.476 | 0.145 |
| Vocalizations | 2.867 | 2.987 | 1.677 | 1.056 | 67 | 0.322 | 0.748 |

* = $p<0.05$
** = $p<0.01$

Table 11.4 Comparisons between means (X) in questionnaire IBQ assessment in Down's syndrome and non-delayed infants at 9 and 12 months

| 9 months | | | | | | | |
|---|---|---|---|---|---|---|---|
| *IBQ* | *X Down's* | *X Non-delayed* | *SD Down's* | *SD Non-delayed* | *D F* | *T* | *Probability* |
| Level of activity | 5.408 | 4.804 | 0.884 | 0.842 | 64 | –2.228 | 0.029* |
| Distress to limitations | 4.118 | 3.961 | 0.622 | 0.783 | 64 | –0.651 | 0.517 |
| Fear | 3.593 | 3.080 | 0.950 | 0.648 | 64 | –2.264 | 0.027* |
| Duration of orientation | 3.993 | 3.344 | 1.115 | 1.060 | 64 | –1.901 | 0.062 |
| Laughter/ Smiling | 4.930 | 4.731 | 0.658 | 0.621 | 64 | –0.994 | 0.324 |
| Soothability | 4.638 | 4.581 | 0.947 | 1.275 | 64 | –0.146 | 0.885 |
| **12 months** | | | | | | | |
| *IBQ* | *X Down's* | *X Non-delayed* | *SD Down's* | *SD Non-delayed* | *D F* | *T* | *Probability* |
| Level of activity | 4.947 | 4.352 | 0.610 | 0.888 | 66 | -2.284 | 0.026* |
| Distress to limitations | 4.159 | 4.024 | 0.508 | 0.925 | 66 | –0.507 | 0.614 |
| Fear | 3.438 | 3.935 | 0.679 | 0.742 | 66 | 2.205 | 0.031* |
| Duration of orientation | 3.979 | 3.533 | 0.525 | 0.905 | 66 | –1.706 | 0.093 |
| Laughter/ Smiling | 4.905 | 4.711 | 0.645 | 0.755 | 66 | –0.854 | 0.396 |
| Soothability | – | – | – | – | – | – | – |

* = $p<0.05$

Our results confirm the existence of individual differences in the temperament of infants with DS. The analysis of behaviour in laboratory conditions has revealed that the characteristics of emotional tone, activity level, attention, social orientation, and vocalization are reliable indicators of the differences among infants with DS at the two periods studied in the development of the child. Similarly, our results suggest that the IBQ is a valid and effective instrument for detecting temperament characteristics in the aforementioned stages of development, i.e., activity level, distress to limitations, duration of orientation, smiling and laughter and soothability. However, DS infants as a group are heterogeneous regarding behavioural characteristics. As is the case for non-delayed infants, a wide range of characteristics and profiles are observed.

As is clear from the analysis of temperament in laboratory conditions, the affective tone of interaction at 9 months correlates with all the other dimensions, and particularly with that of attention. This suggests that infants considered very positive in their environment also contemplate their surroundings for longer periods of time, are also found to be the most active and among those producing more vocalizations. At 12 months, emotional tone continues to be an essential dimension maintaining a close relationship with activity level, attention and vocalization. As we can see, the characteristics of the profile that differentiates the subjects from one another remain in evidence at this second point in development.

Another aspect that confirms the similarities between the group of DS and non-delayed infants is that the different temperament dimensions are grouped in the same way at 9 months, excluding that of vocalization in the DS infants. Practically the same situation exists at 12 months when the dimensions are split into two groups: one, consisting of emotional tone, activity level, and vocalization, and another one consisting of social orientation and attention. Thus, as a group, DS infants undergo a process of development in which the changes in the expression of temperament can be considered as being as much a product of the maturing process and the development of the brain as of the organization of cognitive and self-regulatory capacities (Rothbart and Derryberry 1981).

According to the laboratory results, the temperamental dimensions that show stability at both ages analysed are the following: emotional tone, activity level and vocalization. We can therefore observe that the infants who scored more highly in emotional tone in the first evaluation also did so in the second evaluation. The same thing occurred with the dimensions of activity and vocalization. On the other hand, it is important to emphasize the lack of stability in the dimension of attention. DS infants need more time to evaluate a situation. Therefore, it is not surprising that the lack of stability observed is related to the specific characteristics that its expression has in this population as well as to the processes of change that the maturation and organization of their cognitive capacities have at these ages.

When we analyse the mothers' reports, a stability in all the temperamental dimensions is found in the group of non-delayed infants. The same stability is less general in the DS infants, appearing only in the dimensions of activity level, fear and soothability. As Ganiban *et al.* (1990) have pointed out, the presence of changes in temperament characteristics can reflect as much processes of normal maturation as changes in the parents with respect to the expectations and reactions towards their children.

If, generally speaking, important qualitative differences are not perceived between DS and non-delayed infants as groups at similar levels of development, they may be observed from a quantitative perspective. The results obtained from the laboratory study indicated that the DS infants differ from the group of non-delayed infants in the lower intensity of expression of positive and negative affect, in a greater degree of attention and a lower activity level. These quantitative differences confirm previous findings (Rothbart and Hanson 1983; Gunn *et al.* 1983; Gunn and Berry 1985). Our results suggest, as those of Gunn and Berry (1985), that quantitative differences may exist that are not attributable to cognitive development. Thus, it cannot be maintained that if the level of development in DS infants is controlled, the differences in intensity of response will disappear in relation to non-delayed infants. In short, these differences may have their origin in the sensitivity of the response systems of individuals with DS, hence they may appear less responsive to stimulation than groups of non-delayed children (Thompson *et al.* 1985). This low physiological reaction to new situations is reflected in their approach to and behaviour within their environment. Therefore they may initially appear non-interactive, less approachable but highly attentive.

These quantitative differences do not show up when comparisons between both groups are made by studying the mothers' reports. It is difficult to interpret the two dimensions in which quantitative differences are produced, i.e., activity level and fear. For example, we have observed that activity level appears higher in the group of DS infants than in that of non-delayed infants at 9 months MA. It is probable that the difference in terms of CA has an effect on the general perception of the aforementioned temperament dimension. However, it is surprising that later, at 12 months, the mothers perceive their children as being less active. Furthermore, if we take into account that for the remaining dimensions, excluding fear, the intensity of response is similar to that of the other group of infants, it may be that, among other possible explanations, the mothers have established unrealistic expectations about the response capacity of their children.

## References

Baron J (1972) Temperament profile of children with Down's syndrome. Developmental Medicine and Child Neurology 14: 640–3.

Bayley N (1977) Escalas Bayley de Desarrollo Infantil. Madrid: TEA.

Beeghly M, Perry BW and Cicchetti D (1989) Structural and affective dimensions of play development in young children with Down syndrome. International Journal of Behavioral Development 12: 257–77.

Berger J and Cunningham CC (1986) Aspects of early social smiling by infants with Down's syndrome. Child: Care, Health and Development 12: 13–24.

Berry P, Gunn P and Andrews R (1980) Behavior of Down syndrome infants in a strange situation. American Journal of Mental Deficiency 85: 213–18.

Bridges FA and Cicchetti D (1982) Mothers' ratings of the temperament characteristics of Down syndrome infants. Developmental Psychology 18: 238–44.

Buss AH and Plomin R (1984) Temperament: Early developing personality traits. Hillsdale NJ: Erlbaum.

Candel I and Carranza JA (1993) Características evolutivas de los niños con síndrome de Down en la infancia. In I Candel (Ed) Programa de atención temprana. intervención en niños con síndrome de Down y otros problemas de desarrollo, pp. 54–87. Madrid: CEPE.

Cicchetti D and Serafica FC (1981) Interplay among behavioral systems: Illustrations from the study of attachment, affiliation and wariness in young children with Down's syndrome. Developmental Psychology 17: 36–49.

Cicchetti D and Sroufe LA (1976) The relationship between affective and cognitive development in Down's syndrome infants. Child Development 47: 920–9.

Cicchetti D and Sroufe LA (1978) An organizational view of affect: Illustrations of the study of Down's syndrome infants. In M Lewis and L Rosenblum (Eds) The Development of affect, pp. 309–50. New York: Plenum.

Flórez J (1995) Patología cerebral en el síndrome de Down: aprendizaje y conducta. In J Perera (Ed) Síndrome de Down. Aspectos específicos, pp. 27–52. Barcelona: Masson.

Ganiban J, Wagner S and Cicchetti D (1990) Temperament and Down syndrome. In D Cicchetti and M Beeghly (Eds) Children with Down syndrome. A developmental perspective, pp. 63–100. New York: Cambridge University Press.

Gibson D (1978) Down syndrome. London: Cambridge University Press.

Goldberg S and Marcovitch S (1989) Temperament in developmentally disabled children. In GA Kohnstamm, JE Bates and M Rothbart (Eds) Temperament in childhood, pp. 387–403. New York: Wiley.

Gunn P, Berry P and Andrews S (1983) The temperament of Down syndrome toddlers: A research note. Journal of Child Psychology and Psychiatry 24: 601-5.

Gunn P and Berry P (1985) The temperament of Down's syndrome toddlers and their siblings. Journal of Child Psychology and Psychiatry 26: 973–9.

Kemper TL (1988) Neuropathology of Down syndrome. In L Nadel (Ed) The psychobiology of Down syndrome, pp. 269–89. London: MIT Press.

Lerner J (1993) The influence of child temperamental characteristics on parent behaviors. In T Luster and L Okagaki (Eds) Parenting. An ecological perspective, pp. 101–20. Hillsdale: Eerlbaum.

Loeches A (1988) Discriminación y expresión de emociones en bebés con síndrome de Down. Unpublished doctoral dissertation, Universidad Autónoma, Madrid.

MacTurk RH, Vietze P, McCarthy M, McQuiston S and Yarrow L (1985) The organization of exploratory behavior in Down syndrome and nondelayed infants. Child Development 56: 573–81.

Marcovitch S, Goldberg S, MacGregor D and Lojkasek M (1986) Patterns of temperament variation in three groups of developmentally delayed preschool children: Mother and father ratings. Developmental and Behavioral Pediatrics 7: 247–52.

Matheny L Jr AP and Wilson RS (1981) Developmental tasks and rating scales for the laboratory assessment of infant temperament. Catalog of Selected Documents in Psychology 11, 81 (Manuscript 2643).

Motti F, Cicchetti D and Sroufe LA (1983) From infant affect expression to symbolic play: the coherence of development in Down syndrome children. Child Development 54: 168–75.

Rothbart M (1981) Measurement of temperament in infancy. Child Development 52: 569–78.

Rothbart M and Derryberry D (1981) The development of individual differences in temperament. In M Lamb and AL Brown (Eds) Advances in developmental psychology 1: pp. 37–86. Hillsdale, NJ: Erlbaum.

Rothbart M and Hanson MJ (1983) A caregiver report comparison of temperamental characteristics of Down syndrome and normal infants. Developmental Psychology 19: 766–9.

Sorce J and Emde R (1982) The meaning of infant emotional expressions: regularities in caregiving responses in normal and Down's syndrome infants. Journal of Child Psychology and Psychiatry 23: 145–58.

Thomas A and Chess S (1977) Temperament and Development. New York: Brunner/Mazel.

Thompson R, Cichetta D and MalKin L (1985) The emotional responses of Down syndrome and normal infants in the strange situation: The organization of affective behavior in infants. Developmental Psychology 21: 828–41.

Vaughn BE, Contreras J and Seifer R (1994) Short-term longitudinal study of maternal ratings of temperament in samples of children with Down syndrome and children who are developing normally. American Journal on Mental Retardation 98: 607–18.

Wisniewski KE (1990) Down syndrome children often have brain with maturation delay, retardation of growth and cortical dysgenesis. American Journal of Medical Genetics, Supplement 7: 274–81.

# 12

# Psychiatric Disorders and Behavioural Concerns in Persons with Down's Syndrome

SIEGFRIED M PUESCHEL, BEVERLY MYERS AND MARIA SUSTROVA

## 12.1 Introduction

The first part of this paper will discuss psychiatric disorders as they relate to persons with Down's syndrome (DS). Previous reports will be briefly reviewed and then the results of our investigations shall be presented.

The second part of this paper will focus on behavioural issues in children with DS. The pertinent literature of this topic will be highlighted followed by a description of our studies on behavioural concerns in children with DS.

## 12.2 Psychiatric Disorders

There are only a few reports in the literature pertaining to psychiatric disorders in individuals with DS. In 1965, Menolascino reported his study of children with DS. He found 11 of 86 (13%) children to have psychiatric conditions. A study by Gath and Gumley (1986) revealed that 73 of 193 (38%) children and adolescents with DS had psychiatric disorders.

In adults only one psychiatric survey of individuals with DS has been carried out (Lund 1988). In a study of 324 adults with mental retardation living in the community, Lund reported that 11 of 44 (25%) persons with DS had psychiatric problems.

Our study (Myers and Pueschel 1991) included 425 individuals with DS who are followed as outpatients at the Child Development Center of Rhode Island Hospital. Another 72 persons with DS residing at a nearby state school for individuals with mental retardation were also part of this study. Thus, there were a total of 497 persons with DS enrolled in this project. We examined the medical records of all individuals and obtained demographic data on each patient including age, sex and race. Medical information was recorded such as the presence or absence of congenital heart disease, pulmonary, orthopedic, central nervous system, thyroid, hearing and vision disorders. In particular, psychiatric diagnoses were made based upon psychiatric and psychological evaluations, multidisciplinary reports, and the description of the patients' behavioural and emotional status.

The results of this investigation (see Table 12.1) showed that there were 261 individuals below the age of 20 years and 164 persons aged 20 years and older from the Child Development Center in addition to the 72 older persons from the state school. The average age of the study population was 19.4 years, ranging from 1 to 72 years. There were 288 males and 209 females. Most of the subjects were white (95%) and there were only a few individuals with Down's syndrome of other races. Ninety per cent of the study population of whom chromosome analyses were available had trisomy 21, 4% had translocations, and 6% had mosaicism Down's syndrome. One hundred and ten of 497 individuals with DS (22.1%) had various forms of psychiatric disorders. There were 46 patients below the age of 20 years and 64 persons 20 years and older with psychiatric disorders. The younger age group included persons with disruptive behaviours such as attention deficit problems, conduct/oppositional and aggressive behaviours, anxiety disorders and repetitive behaviours. Similar behaviours were also observed in some adults. However, in addition, a significant number of these older patients had major depressive disorders. Some state school residents were thought to have dementia.

When we compare the results of our investigations with those of previous studies, we observe that children with DS below the age of 10 years in our cohort had a similar prevalence of psychiatric disorders (14.7%) as Menolascino's outpatient population of whom 13% had psychiatric disorders (Menolascino 1965). However, Menolascino's (1970) institutionalized population and also Gath and Gumley's (1986) patients revealed a markedly higher prevalence of psychiatric disorders, namely 37% and 38% respectively.

The prevalence of psychiatric disorders of patients with DS syndrome followed at the Child Development Center of Rhode Island Hospital who are 20 years and older is similar to that of Lund's (1988) population. Lund observed that 25% of adults with DS had psychiatric disorders, and we found such psychiatric conditions in 25.6%. When we compare the prevalence of psychiatric disorders in persons with DS with that of other populations with mental retardation due to a different etiology, psychiatric disorders in the latter group were reported to be significantly higher (32% to 59% by Lund 1988; 30%, by Rutter *et al.* 1970). Thus, persons with DS may have a lower risk for psychiatric disor-

Table 12.1 Results of Myers and Pueshel's (1991) study

| | CDC* Patients <20 years | | CDC Patients ≥20 years | | State School Residents | | Total | |
|---|---|---|---|---|---|---|---|---|
| Disruptive disorders | | | | | | | | |
| Attention deflict disorder | 16 | 6.1% | 4 | 2.4% | 1 | 1.3% | 21 | 4.2% |
| Conduct/oppositional disorder | 14 | 5.4% | 3 | 1.8% | 1 | 1.3% | 18 | 3.6% |
| Aggressive behaviour | 17 | 6.5% | 10 | 6.1% | 9 | 1.2% | 36 | 7.2% |
| Anxiety disorders | | | | | | | | |
| Phobias | 4 | 1.5% | 1 | 0.6% | | | 5 | 1% |
| Obsessive-compulsive behaviour | | | 1 | 0.6% | 3 | 4.1% | 4 | 0.8% |
| Conversion disorder | | | 1 | 0.6% | | | | |
| Gastrointestinal disorders | | | | | | | | |
| Eating problems | 2 | 0.8% | 3 | 1.8% | 1 | 1.3% | 6 | 1.2% |
| Elimination difficulties | 4 | 1.5% | 1 | 0.6% | 3 | 4.1% | 8 | 1.6% |
| Repetitive behaviours | | | | | | | | |
| Tourette syndrome | 1 | 0.4% | 2 | 1.2% | | | 3 | 0.6% |
| Stereotypic behaviour | 7 | 2.7% | 7 | 4.3% | | | 14 | 2.8% |
| Self-injurious behaviour | 2 | 0.8% | 2 | 1.2% | 4 | 5.5% | 8 | 1.6% |
| Affective disorders | | | | | | | | |
| Major depressive disorders | | | 10 | 6.1% | | | 10 | 2% |
| Manic depressive disorders | | | 1 | 0.6% | | | 1 | 0.2% |
| Organic affective syndromes | | | | | 1 | 1.3% | 1 | 0.2% |
| Others | | | | | | | | |
| Dementias | | | 1 | 0.6% | 5 | 6.1% | 6 | 1.1% |
| Paraphilias | | | 3 | 1.2% | | | 3 | 0.6% |
| Psychosis | | | 1 | 0.6% | | | 1 | 0.2% |
| Schizophrenia | | | 0 | 0% | 0 | 0% | 0 | 0% |
| Autism | 3 | 1.1% | 2 | 1.2% | | | 5 | 1% |
| TOTAL** | 46 | 17.6% | 42 | 25.6% | 22 | 30.5% | 110 | 22.1% |

* Child Center Development

** Some patients have more than one psychiatric disorder

ders than individuals with mental retardation who do not have this chromosome disorder.

The frequency of specific psychiatric diagnoses in our population of children with DS was contrasted with that of studies by Menolascino (1965, 1970) and Gath and Gumley (1986). There was a significant difference with respect to the prevalence of autism. We only observed 1% of 497 patients with DS to have autism, whereas Gath and Gumley (1986) reported 10%, and Lund (1988) found 11.3% of patients with autism.

Similarly, a discrepancy of the frequency of attention deficit disorders was noted. We observed 6.1% of children and adolescents below the age of 20 years with attention deficit disorder, whereas Green *et al.* (1989) reported attention deficit disorders at a much high frequency (36%). Also, self-injurious behaviour and stereotypic movements were observed at a lower frequency in our study population, 1.6% and 2.8% respectively. In individuals with mental retardation due to other etiology, such behaviours were observed more often (Oliver *et al.* 1987).

Our investigations as well as those of others demonstrated that there is an increased vulnerability to depression in adults with DS. We found that 6.1% of our adult population had depressive disorders. Keegan *et al.* (1974) and Szymanski and Biederman (1984) also observed a slightly higher prevalence of major depressive disorders in people with DS when compared with a control population. However, Lund (1988) did not find any patients with depression among 44 individuals with DS. The presence of depressive disorders in adults with DS may be due to specific environmental stressors, genetic factors, and/or represent the early stages of a dementing process.

A wide range of other psychopathology in adults with DS was noted including obsessive compulsive disorders, anorexia nervosa, phobias, conversion reactions, paraphilias, Tourette syndrome and eating disorders. The frequency of these disorders are detailed in Table 12.1. Although other authors had observed schizophrenia among persons with DS (Menolascino 1970), we did not find any individual in our study with classical signs of schizophrenia. Moreover, there was no patient in our study with personality disorders, substance abuse, sleep disorders, adjustment reactions and alcoholism.

Thus, we observed a broad range of psychopathology in our study population of nearly 500 persons with DS. As mentioned above, the overall prevalence of psychiatric disorders of 22.1% is less than that observed in other mentally retarded people of different etiology. Children with DS are more likely to exhibit disruptive disorders including attention deficit problems, conduct/oppositional disorders and aggressive behaviours. Adults with DS living in the community display, in addition, paraphilias and, often, major depressive disorders. Dementia was more prevalent in the state school population which was also found in a recent study by Haveman *et al.* (1994).

## 12.3 Behavioural Observations in Persons with Down's Syndrome

During the past few decades, there has been a growing interest in the behaviour of children with developmental disabilities. Carr and Hewitt (1982) reported that 22% of mothers of 11-year-old youngsters with DS worried about their children's behaviour. Gath and Gumley (1986) described various behaviour problems in 193 children with DS. They found that 38% of them had significant behaviour disorders. The authors noted that conduct disorders were present more often in children with DS than in other children.

Reviewing the literature on behaviour in persons with DS, many authors (Benda 1946; Domino 1965; Gibbs and Thorpe 1983) have described specific behavioural traits in children with DS, such as good-tempered, affectionate, placid, stubborn, withdrawn and defiant behaviours. However, as early as 1953, Blacketter-Simmonds reported that the social performance of persons with DS did not fit the stereotype and was not homogeneous. In 1972, Baron reported that the behaviour of children with DS was similar to that of the 'normal' population when mental age was taken into account. Also, other investigators including Robinson and Robinson (1976), Bridges and Cicchetti (1982), Gunn *et al.* (1983), and Rodgers (1987) indicated that this old stereotype as described above is probably incorrect and that children with DS have the same range of personality and behavioural attributes as seen in other children who do not have this chromosome disorder. A recent study by Cuskelly and Dadds (1992) deals with behaviour problems in children with DS. The authors noted that children with DS were reported to display more problem behaviours and showed significantly more attentional problems than their siblings.

In our studies (Pueschel *et al.* 1991; Pueschel and Myers 1994), 40 children with DS and their families were enrolled. We employed the following instruments: the *Achenbach Child Behavior Checklist,* the *Family Environmental Scale,* and the *Temperament Assessment Battery for Children*.

The *Achenbach Child Behavior Checklist* is designed to record, in a standardized form, behavioural attributes and competencies of children between the ages of 4 and 16 years (Achenbach and Edelbrock 1983). There are two broad-band groupings in all sex/age groups referred to by Achenbach as the internalizing-externalizing dichotomy.

The *Family Environmental Scale* is designed to measure the social characteristics of all types of families (Moss and Moss 1984). The instrument's 10 subscales are supposed to assess three major domains: *relationship, personal growth*, and *system maintenance.* The relationship dimension is measured by the cohesion, expressiveness and conflict subscales. The personal growth dimension encompasses the independence, achievement orientation, intellectual/cultural orientation, active-recreational, and moral/religious emphasis subscales. The system maintenance dimension comprises the organization and control subscales (Moss and Moss 1984).

The *Temperament Assessment Battery for Children* focuses on information on the children's behaviour in different situations (Martin 1988).

This scale consists of three different rating scales that measure basic personality/behavioural dimensions of young children. The six basic behaviours that are measured on this scale include activity, adaptability, approach/withdrawal, emotional intensity, distractibility and persistence.

Using the *Achenbach Child Behavior Checklist*, we did not find any significant difference between the study and control group with regard to the internalizing scores obtained from both parents and teachers responses. However, statistically significant differences were observed between study and control groups on externalizing and total scores from both teachers' and parents' responses.

Further analysis of our data, using Achenbach's taxonomy of profile pattern for both boys and girls revealed a 'hyperactive' profile as shown in Figures 12.1 and 12.2 respectively. There was a statistically significant difference ($p < 0.001$) comparing study and control groups for both boys and girls.

Figure 12.3 shows the mean scores of individual items in the 'hyperactive' category of children with DS and those of control children. When we engaged in an item analysis of the 'hyperactive' category, we found that it is heavily weighted by positive responses to such statements 'acts too young for his/her age,' 'can't concentrate,' 'can't pay attention for long,' 'impulsive, or acts without thinking,' and particularly 'speech problems.' Although the majority of scores were made up of these items, some of the children (9 out of 16 boys and 5 out of 12 girls) indeed exhibited hyperactive behaviours. In general, parents indicated that their child with DS was more active than the sibling in the control group. Thus, our data are in sharp contrast to previous reports that stereotyped the child with DS as placid, inactive and lethargic.

When we compared the scores on individual items between the children with DS and those obtained from the control children, significant differences were observed on items 'acts too young for his/her age,' 'speech problems,' 'trouble sleeping,' 'can't concentrate,' 'demands a lot of attention,' 'clings to adult or dependent,' and 'stubborn, sullen, or irritable'. Although many parents of our children with DS reported that their child was stubborn, it is possible that this 'stereotypic' behaviour is not necessarily the result of a true observation, but rather a self-fulfilling prophecy since many parents had been told previously that they should expect their child with DS to be stubborn.

It is of note that the item analysis of most responses in the *Achenbach Child Behavior Checklist* did not reveal any significant differences between the study and control populations. Thus, most of the behaviours recorded compare well with other children who do not have DS.

The *Family Environmental Scale* profiles indicated on the average high scores in cohesion, expressiveness, achievement, moral/religious emphasis, and organization, as shown in Figure 12.4. The above-

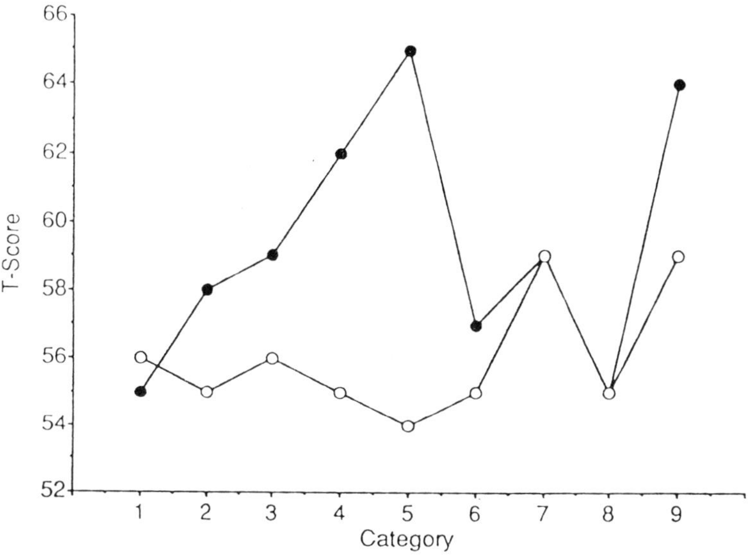


*Figure 12.1* Mean values of categories 1–9 of the *Achenbach Child Behavior Checklist* of boys with Down's syndrome ($n$=16) ( ● ) and boys of the control group ($n$=12) ( ○ ): (1) 'schizoid or anxious'; (2) 'depressed'; (3) 'uncommunicative'; (4) 'obsessive–compulsive'; (5) 'somatic complaints'; (6) 'social withdrawal'; (7) 'hyperactive'; (8) 'aggressive'; and (9) 'delinquent'.

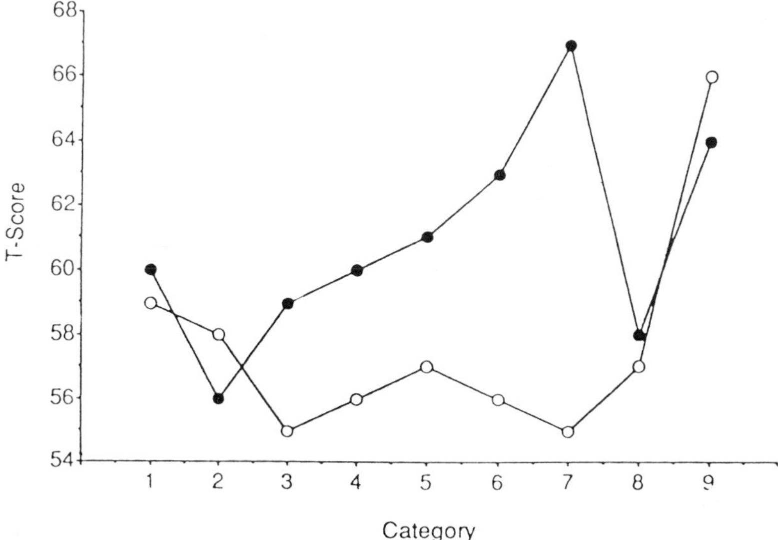


*Figure 12.2* Mean values of categories 1–9 of the *Achenbach Child Behavior Checklist* of girls with Down's syndrome ($n$= 12) ( ● ) and girls of the control group ($n$ = 10) ( ○ ): (1) 'depressed'; (2) 'social withdrawal'; (3) 'somatic complaints'; (4) 'schizoid–obsessive'; (5) 'hyperactive'; (6) 'sex problem'; (7) 'delinquent'; (8) 'aggressive'; and (9) 'cruel'.

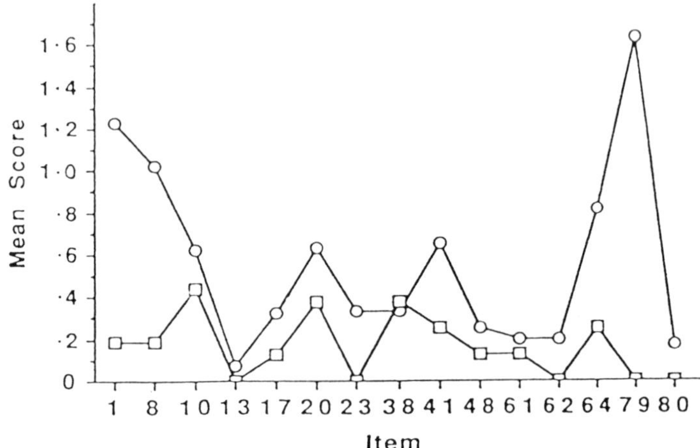


*Figure 12.3* Mean scores of individual items of the 'hyperactive' category of boys and girls with Down's syndrome (n=28) ( ● ) and boys and girls in the control group (n=22) ( ○ ). The following items show a statistically significant difference between individuals with Down's syndrome and those in the control group: (1) 'acts too young, for his/her age'; (8) 'can't concentrate'; (23) 'is disobedient at school'; (41) 'impulsive or acts without thinking'; (64) 'prefers playing with younger children'; and (79) 'speech problems'.

average scores on both cohesion and expressiveness indicate a high degree of commitment and support family members provide for one another as well as the extent to which family members are encouraged to express their feelings. Hence, most families participating in this study are relationship-oriented. They often answered affirmatively statements such as 'we really get along well with each other,' 'we put a lot of energy into what we do at home,' and 'we tell each other about our personal problems.' The average family in this study is also achievement-oriented as demonstrated by a high mean achievement score. Parents answered the following statements affirmatively: 'we always strive to do things a little bit better the next time,' and 'getting ahead in life is very important to our family.' There were also high mean values in the moral/religious and organization categories as parents often answered 'true' to statements such as 'family members have strict ideas about what is right and wrong,' and 'we believe there are some things you just have to take on faith.'

The *Temperament Assessment Battery for Children* profiles as reported by parents and teachers are very similar except for the categories in distractibility where significantly higher scores were reported

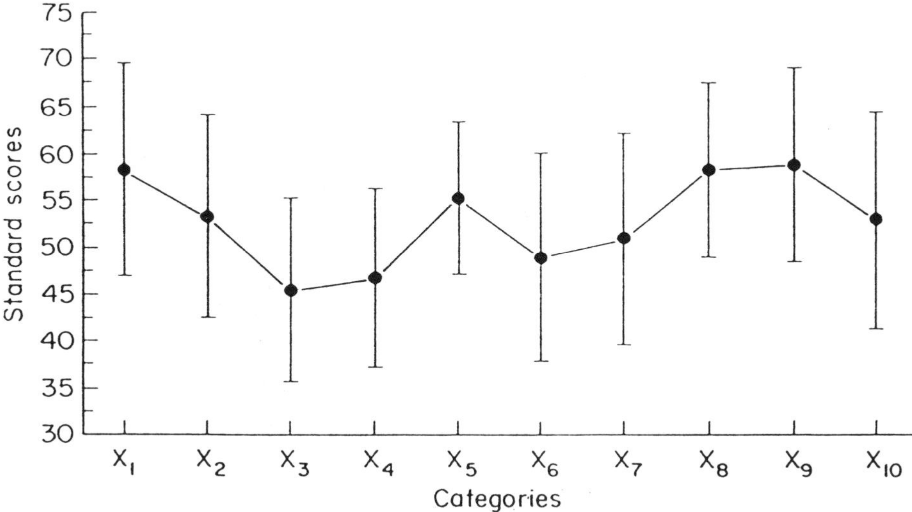


*Figure 12.4* Means and standard deviations of the Family Environment Scale Profile ($X_1$=Cohesion; $X_2$=Expressiveness; $X_3$=Conflict; $X_4$ = Independence; $X_5$=Achievement; $X_6$=Intellectual–cultural; $X_7$=Active–Recreational; $X_8$= Moral–Religious; $X_9$=Organization; X10=Control).

by teachers than by parents (see Figure 12.5). On the *Temperament Assessment Battery for Children,* individuals with DS displayed slightly higher scores than their siblings in all categories except in the emotional intensity and persistence categories; however, statistical significance only in the category approach/withdrawal was reached. This indicated that children with DS are more socially engaging and enjoy new activities. Parents often mentioned that 'the child immediately gets involved in new learning situations' and 'the child plunges into new activities and situations without hesitation.'

Contrasting the *Temperament Assessment Battery for Children* scores and those obtained from the *Family Environmental Scale,* significant positive correlations were found between expressiveness and distractibility ($p$= 0.0181), expressiveness and persistence ($p$ = 0.0189); and a significant negative correlation between expressiveness and activity ($p$ = 0.0395) and control and distractibility ($p$ = 0.029).

The dual investigation of family milieu (*Family Environment Scale)* and behavioural aspects (*Temperament Assessment Battery for Children*), not only provide some insight into the home environment where children with DS are raised, but also permits the study of their temperament profile in such settings. Thus, correlations of specific behaviours obtained from the *Temperament Assessment Battery for Children* with certain environmental conditions can be investigated.

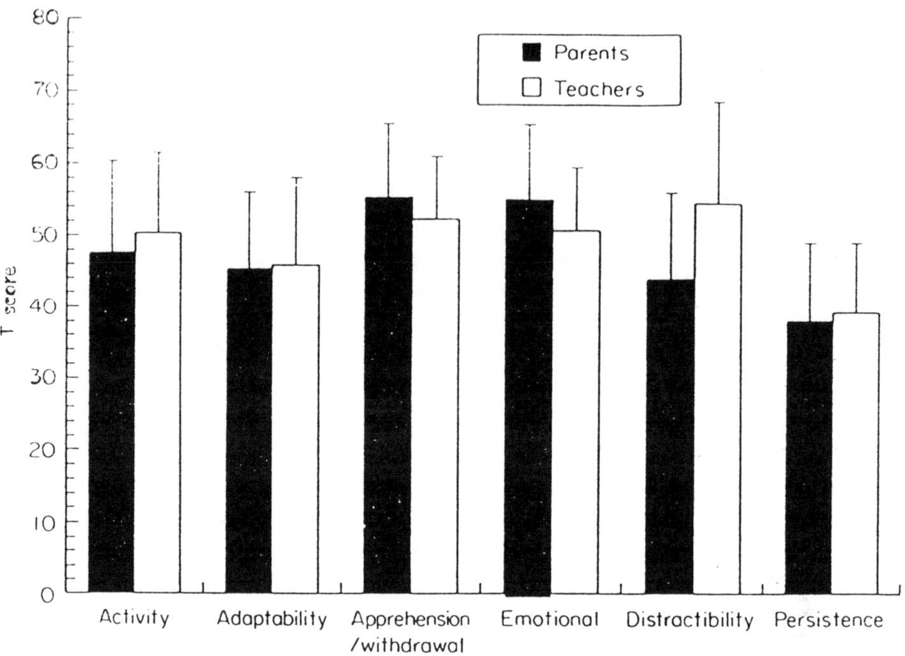


*Figure 12.5* Means and standard deviations of the results of temperament assessment of persons with Down's syndrome as reported by parents and teachers.

In summary, our studies on behaviour, temperament and environmental factors indicate that children with DS are more similar to their brothers and sisters and other children in the community than they are different. When the behavioural data were scored a 'hyperactive' profile pattern emerged. The average family in this study had good interpersonal relationships, could express its feelings directly, is achievement oriented, emphasizes ethical values, and places importance on family organization. Moreover, we found that children with DS are more socially engaging than their siblings, yet the latter group adjusts more easily to new situations and – as expected – is superior to their brothers and sisters with DS in solving difficult learning problems.

It is our contention that up-to-date information on environmental aspects, behavioural and temperamental concerns on children with DS should be obtained and analysed. Only carefully controlled studies where strengths and weaknesses of children's behaviours are identified will permit appropriate remediation. The person with DS is expected to display behaviours that are generally socially acceptable as a prerequisite for optimal functioning in society, whether in the educational setting, in employment situations, or in recreational activities.

# References

Achenbach TM and Edelbrock S (1983) Manual for the Child Behavior Checklist and Revised Child Behavior Profile. Cincinnati OH: Queen City Printers.

Baron J (1972) Temperament profile of children with DS. Developmental Medicine and Child Neurology 14: 640–3.

Benda CE (1946) Mongolism and cretinism. New York: Grune and Stratton.

Berry P, Gunn P and Andrews RJ (1980) Behavior of Down syndrome infants in a strange situation. American Journal of Mental Deficiency 85: 213–18.

Blacketter-Simmonds DA (1953) An investigation into the supposed differences existing between mongols and other mentally defective subjects with regard to certain psychological traits. Journal of Mental Science 99: 702–19.

Bridges FA and Cicchetti D (1982) Mothers' ratings of the temperament characteristics of Down syndrome infants. Developmental Psychology 18: 238–44.

Carr J and Hewitt S (1982) Children with Down's syndrome growing up. Association for Child Psychology and Psychiatry News 10: 43.

Cuskelly M and Dadds M (1992) Behavioral problems in children with Down's syndrome and their siblings. Journal of Child Psychology and Psychiatry 33: 749–61.

Domino G (1965) Personality traits in institutionalized mongoloids. American Journal of Mental Deficiency 69: 568–70.

Gath A and Gumley D (1986) Behavior problems in retarded children with special reference to Down's syndrome. British Journal of Psychiatry 149: 156–61.

Gibbs MV and Thorpe JG (1983) Personality stereotype of noninstitutionalized Down syndrome children. American Journal of Mental Deficiency 87: 601–5.

Green JM, Dennis J and Bennets LA (1989) Attention disorder in a group of young Down's syndrome children. Journal of Mental Deficiency Research 33: 105–22.

Gunn P, Berry P and Andrews JJ (1983) The temperament of Down's syndrome toddlers: a research note. Journal of Child Psychology and Psychiatry 24: 601–5.

Haveman MJ, Maaskant MA, Van Schrojenstein Lantman HM, Urlings HIJ and Kessels AGH (1994) Mental health problems in elderly people with and without Down's syndrome. Journal of Intellectual Disability Research 38: 341–55.

Keegan DL, Pettigrew A and Parker A (1974) Psychosis in Down's syndrome treated with amitriptyline. Canadian Medical Association Journal 110: 1128–33.

Lund J (1988) Psychiatric aspects of Down's syndrome. Acta Psychiatrica Scandinavia 78: 369–74.

Martin RP (1988) Temperament assessment battery for children. Brandon VT: Clinical Psychology Publishing Co Inc.

Menolascino FL (1965) Psychiatric aspects of mongolism. American Journal of Mental Deficiency 69: 653–66.

Menolascino FL (1970) Down's syndrome: Clinical and psychiatric finding in an institutionalized sample. In FJ Menolascino (Ed) Psychiatric approaches to mental retardation. New York: Basic Books.

Moss RH and Moss BS (1984) Family Environmental Scale Manual. Palo Alto CA: Consulting Psychologists Press.

Myers BA and Pueschel SM (1991) Psychiatric disorders in persons with Down's syndrome. The Journal of Nervous and Mental Disease 179: 609–13.

Oliver C, Murphy GH and Corbett JA (1987) Self-injurious behavior in people with mental handicaps: A total population study. Journal of Mental Deficiency Research 31: 147–62.

Pueschel SM, Bernier JC and Pezzullo JC (1991) Behavioral observations in children with Down's syndrome. Journal of Mental Deficiency Research 35: 502–11.

Pueschel SM and Myers BA (1994) Environmental and temperament assessments of children with Down's syndrome. Journal of Intellectual Disability Research 38: 195–202.

Robinson NM and Robinson HB (1976) The mentally retarded child: A psychological approach. New York: McGraw-Hill.

Rodgers C (1987) Maternal support for the Down's syndrome stereotype: the effect of direct experience of the conditions. Journal of Mental Deficiency Research 31: 271–8.

Rutter M, Graham P and Yule W (1970) A neuropsychiatric study in childhood. London: Heinemann .

Szymanski LS (1980) Psychiatric diagnosis of retarded persons. In LS Szymanski and PE Tanguay (Eds) Emotional disorders of mentally retarded persons, pp.48–67. Baltimore MD: University Press.

Szymanski LS and Biederman J (1984) Depression and anorexia nervosa of persons with Down Syndrome. American Journal of Mental Deficiency 89: 246–251.

# 13
# Psychosexual Behaviour, Sexuality and Management Issues in Individuals with Down's Syndrome

DON C. VAN DYKE, DIANNE M. McBRIEN, AND PHILIP J. MATTHEIS

## 13.1 Introduction

The image of the individual with Down's syndrome has changed drastically over the past three decades. The gulf between the routinely institutionalized 'Down's syndrome' baby of the 1960s and the dialogue of two males with DS in *Count Us In* is thankfully wide (Kingsley and Levitz 1994). Improved interdisciplinary and preventive medical management of DS, combined with legislative requirements for appropriate education of the disabled, and with an enlightened societal perspective on the developmentally disabled, have enhanced the outlook for participation in careers, social life and community integration.

As individuals with DS take their place in the community, some may be expected to assume some of the sexual roles that the non-disabled population now takes for granted: lover, spouse, parent. Only recently the repeal of local law prohibiting or impeding marriage of mentally disabled individuals attests to the societal ignorance surrounding the sexuality of these individuals. Their residential settings were often sex-segregated, with little opportunity for outside socialization. And while episodes of the TV show *Life Goes On* showed Corky and his girlfriend Andrea – also a young adult with DS – date and eventually elope, there are no scenes depicting romantic evenings in bed, or hinting at the possibility of children. Clearly, sexual, reproductive and emotional concerns in Down's syndrome now need to be addressed by caregivers serving this population.

The beginning of this chapter will be a discussion of the general medical aspects of sexuality in Down's syndrome, including puberty and fertility issues. Later in the chapter, we will explore common attitudes toward sexuality and related behaviours – both by caregivers (including parents) and by individuals with DS. Educational programmes designed to safeguard this sexually vulnerable population will also be discussed.

This chapter will also address the topics of marriage, pregnancy and parenting, and how caregivers may support and optimize these life phases. Contraception and prevention of sexually transmitted diseases require anticipatory guidance and care both similar and different to those in the non-disabled population. The need for modifications and flexibility based on the individual's cognitive status, compliance and health status will be reviewed.

## 13.2 Medical Aspects of Sexuality

### 13.2.1 Male

Most males with DS are sterile (Coleman 1992). Multiple etiologies have been proposed. Studies by Stearns *et al.* in 1960 reported a reduced sperm count. A study by Benda in 1969 noted a lack of mature sperm. Spermatogenetic arrest has been noted by some authors (Stearns *et al.* 1960; McCoy 1991; Pueschel and Bier 1992). While some authors have not observed spermatogenetic arrest, others have noted oligospermia (Pueschel and Bier 1992). Some authors have suggested that germ cell trisomy may affect sperm viability in these males (Pueschel and Bier 1992). The 1989 case report of Sheridan *et al.* of a male child without DS fathered by a man with DS is consistent with germ cell mosaicism commonly found in the gonadal tissue of individuals with trisomy 21 (Sheridan *et al.* 1989).

The study by Pueschel *et al.* (1985) of adolescent males reported no significant difference in the development of secondary sexual characteristics from those of normal adolescent males, with no significant differences in genital size between these two groups. Follicle stimulating hormone (FSH) and luteinizing hormone (LH) levels have been studied by a number of investigators and parallel the hormonal data of male adolescents without DS undergoing sexual maturation (McCoy 1991; Pueschel and Bier 1992; Pueschel *et al.* 1985; Hsiang *et al.* 1987). Minor urogenital abnormalities have been reported in males with DS (Smith and Berg 1976): Smith and Berg reported an increased incidence of cryptorchidism. Out of 91 males with DS studied by Lang *et al.* (1986), 11 were noted to have an apparent double urethral orifice consistent with coronal hypospadias.

In summary, the onset and rate of puberty in adolescent males is similar to those of their counterparts without DS. While most males are sterile, the etiology of sterility has not been well defined. The genitalia appear to be of normal or slightly below normal size. Urogenital anomalies, including cryptorchidism and hypospadias, have been reported.

### 13.2.2 Female

Most young women with DS experience menarche at roughly the same age as their peers without DS. While previous studies described relatively late menarche, more recent work shows a mean menarchal age of 13.6 years which does not differ significantly from the non-Down's syndrome control mean of 13.5 years. Menses appear to be regular, with a mean cycle length of 28.3 days (Goldstein 1988). Hsiang *et al.* reported elevated mean serum LH and FSH in 14 postpubertal females with DS; they propose an increased incidence of primary gonadal dysfunction in women with DS (Hsiang *et al.* 1987). Peak values of basal body temperature curves, however, have suggested ovulation to occur in a significant number (88.5%) of women with DS (Scola and Pueschel 1992). Women with DS have significant fertility, and births of both chromosomally normal and trisomic infants have been reported (Bovicelli *et al.* 1982). Both precocious and delayed puberty have been reported in females with DS (Coleman 1992). In either instance, medical evaluation with special attention to thyroid, gastrointestinal and cardiac function is warranted.

In summary, females with DS generally achieve pubertal milestones with normal timing and sequence. While there may be an increased incidence of primary gonadal dysfunction, females with DS are usually presumed fertile. Precocious puberty or delayed puberty are not normal findings in this population, and must be evaluated with the DS-related disease complex in mind.

## 13.3 Masturbation

Masturbation is a form of self-stimulation usually involving the genitals. Masturbation may be solitary or mutual; it may be the primary form of self-gratification or the prelude to sexual intercourse (Monat-Haller 1992). Masturbation also can occur as a self-injurious behaviour, most notably in severely to profoundly mentally retarded individuals; it may be, but rarely is, accompanied by genital tissue injury.

Some authors report a 40% incidence of regular masturbation in males with DS; a group of female counterparts had an incidence of 52% (Coleman 1992). Genital exposure, public masturbation, and fantasies have been described. The literature suggests that these behaviours are not more common in the Down's syndrome group than in the general population (Myers and Pueschel 1991).

Deriving emotional and physical satisfaction from sexual life, a difficult task under the best of circumstances, may be fraught with problems for the adolescent and young adult with DS. The young individual's emerging sexuality may disturb parents and caretakers, who may view this normal phase as a potential menace. Sexually transmitted disease and unwanted pregnancy, the twin threats of adolescent sexual culture, may loom even larger to concerned adults when the teenager in question has a cognitive disability. Parents, caregivers and educators are rightfully concerned about this population's sexual vulnerability.

## 13.4 Sexual Behaviour

The individual with DS engaging in sexual behaviour may encounter considerable prejudice. The sex-segregated living arrangements and lack of available social outlets for the mentally disabled demonstrate a societal denial of this group's sexuality (Edwards 1988). The collective memory of the passive, sweet-natured, institutional denizen with DS tends to die hard; the idea that this same group shares our instincts may shame and frighten some. Parents may find it difficult to accept their children as sexual beings. As Nigro observes:

> The parents of a handicapped child...may be dealing with a dependent person whose relationship to the parents continues to be childlike in many respects, whose time and activities continue to be family-centred, whose peer relationships are limited...Indeed, many parents of handicapped children never acknowledged their potential adulthood (and eventually their actual adulthood), so it is not hard to understand their reluctance to perceive sexual needs or their inability to prepare themselves and their child for a healthy, happy, sexual future. (Nigro 1975, p.126)

Counselling regarding appropriate sexual and social behaviours can ease the transition of young DS individuals into adulthood. A wonderfully specific example of such intervention is recalled by Jason Kingsley and Mitchell Levitz, two young men with DS, in their book *Count Us In*:

> When she says no to (inappropriate touching)...that's it. I'll just stop immediately before I get into trouble. What I'm going to do. When I approach a girl like this, I'll say to myself immediately, 'Stop, danger, caution, trouble, touch trouble'. (Kingsley and Levitz 1994, p.68)

## 13.5 Sexual Abuse

Sexual abuse experts recognize that mentally disabled children and adults are particularly vulnerable to sexual exploitation and abuse (Schwab 1992). These individuals, therefore, require individualized education when appropriate, as well as screening for evidence of sexual abuse as part of the routine physical examination. Diligence is warranted; in a 1990 study of 35 mentally retarded women by Elvik *et al.*, 37% demonstrated findings consistent with vaginal penetration. The prevalence of sexual abuse in males is not known. In a review by Schor of 87 non-institutionalized mentally retarded individuals, sexual intercourse had occurred in 50% of those who were mildly mentally retarded with less frequency of sexual intercourse noted in those who were moderately or severely retarded. In the same population, rape or incest had occurred in 33% of those who were mildly retarded and 25% of those who were moderately retarded, with many repeat cases noted (Schor 1987).

A number of factors place the retarded young person at risk for sexual maltreatment. His or her life is often isolated; his or her peer group is usually small, with limited resources for mutual support; the living situation involves multiple, often transient caretakers, particularly in the group home or sheltered apartment environment. Schor suggests that: '...some paedophiles...may be especially attracted to the childlike behaviours of certain retarded adolescents. Others may take satisfaction in engaging in adult sexual activities without having to interact otherwise on an adult level'. (Schor 1987, p.47.)

A disabled person's emotional history also places him or her at risk for sexual abuse. His or her loneliness and frustration at being 'different' may leave him or her eager to accept any form of individual attention. 'Their increased difficulties in achieving age-appropriate goals may heighten their sense of frustration and despair. They often are more easily led and may have greater desire to please caregivers than would a typical teenager. Previous rejections and isolation may increase their responsiveness to attention and affection, contributing to their heightened vulnerability.' (Schor 1987, p.54.)

## 13.6 Sexuality and Sex: Education

Human beings are by definition sexual beings. Each has a unique potential experience of sexuality that may or may not include intercourse. A physical or mental disability does not preclude the desire or ability to obtain sexual gratification or intimacy.

The current educational trend towards early and open sex education should include students with DS. While individuals with DS possess the right to emotionally satisfying and culturally appropriate sexual behaviour, they also need counselling and support services that can both encourage such behaviour and promote good sexual decision-making. The significant range of cognitive levels, learning styles, living and work arrangements, and health problems in the Down's syndrome population requires an individualized approach to sexuality and sex education.

Educational programmes to promote good sexual decision-making have been implemented in many centres. Given the wide range of intellectual ability even within the Down's syndrome population, educators obviously must individualize such plans, as appropriate, to each person's cognitive status. One popular teaching method is the *Circles Concept* (see Figure 13.1), a paradigm of physical and emotional distance (Walker-Hirsch and Champagne 1992). Each circle in a concentric design represents a particular personal relationship and an appropriate corresponding

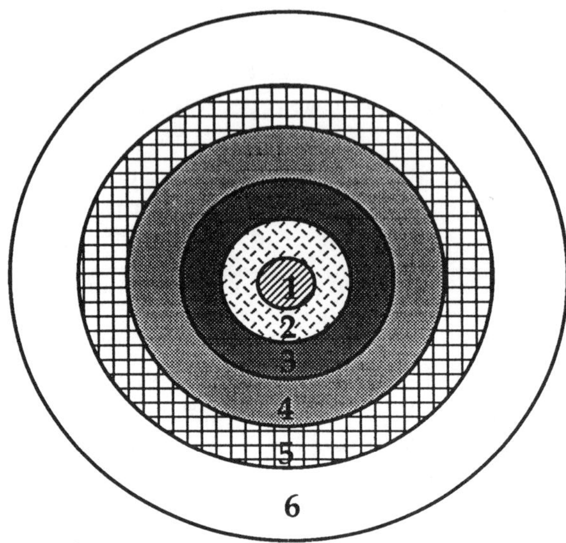


1. Private Circle
2. Hug Circle
3. Far Away Circle
4. Handshake Circle
5. Wave Circle
6. Stranger Circle

*Figure 13.1* Circles concept (Walker-Hirsch L and Champagne MP (1992) Circles III: Safer ways. In AC Crocker, HJ Cohen and TA Kastner (Eds) HIV infection and developmental disabilities, p. 149. Baltimore, MD: Brooks. Reprinted with permission from Paul H Brooks Publishing Co, PO Box 10624. Baltimore, Maryland 21285-0624)

degree of physical intimacy; the individual forms the centre. Students learn, for example, that strangers occupy the 'Stranger Space' (circle 6) and are not supposed to touch them. The subtleties of 'inner circle' relationships are emphasized as well. Friends and extended family members, for example, belong in the 'Far Away' Circle (circle 3). Students learn here that, 'Sometimes a friend may want to be closer to you than you want. You just explain to your friend and say "STOP!"'(Walker-Hirsch and Champagne 1992).

Individuals with DS who have severe cognitive and/or language impairment may be better suited to learn from the 'good touch/bad touch' model commonly used in elementary school abuse prevention programmes. Students learn which body parts may appropriately be touched, as well as which situations are likely to promote 'bad touch' (Monat-Haller 1992). Of course, such training does not obviate the need for conscientious monitoring by mandated reporters involved with the Down's syndrome population (Schor 1987).

# 13.7 Sexuality and Family Life for the Individual with Down's Syndrome

### 13.7.1 Pregnancy

Women with DS can conceive and carry a pregnancy to term. While their fertility seems to be relatively decreased (Hsiang *et al.*'s study demonstrated commonly elevated serum gonadotropin levels consistent with primary ovarian dysfunction) live births both with and without DS have been described (Hsiang *et al.* 1987). An earlier review noted that 30 pregnancies in women with DS, which were fathered by men without DS, resulted in 10 infants with DS, 18 without DS including one set of twins, and 3 spontaneous abortions. The infants without DS demonstrated a greater than average number of congenital anomalies (Bovicelli *et al.* 1982). A more recent review of the series by Rani *et al.* of 31 pregnancies of women with DS added one normal pregnancy outcome to this series (Rani *et al.* 1990).

Until recently, men with DS were considered to be sterile (Smith and Berg 1976). A 1989 report by Sheridan *et al.*, however, describes a 46 XY male infant born to a man with DS and a woman without DS . The man's paternity was established by both cytogenetic and DNA studies (Sheridan *et al.* 1989).

### 13.7.2 Marriage

A study by Edgerton (1993) suggested that, as in many marriages in the general population, the marriages of mentally disabled persons tend to be complementary. In short, the skills of one partner compensate for the other's weaknesses, and vice versa. It is of note that in the 1988 study by Koller, Richardson and Katz of marriages among mentally disabled individuals, none of the partners were severely disabled. Most of his married subjects were mildly disabled and demonstrated higher IQs than the rest of the mildly disabled segment of the general population. While mentally disabled women exhibited more marital problems than women in the general population, almost half of the disabled female subjects appeared to be functioning well in their marriages. No significant differences in marital problem rates were noted between mentally disabled men and 'normal' controls. The most troubled marriages seemed to be those in which both partners were mentally disabled (Koller *et al.* 1988). In light of the United States' current divorce rate of over 50%, the failure rate of marriages with one disabled partner may not necessarily represent unusual marital risk.

Little data exists on individuals with DS who marry. A survey by Edwards (1988) described 38 married persons with DS. Of these subjects, 35 were female; all but one had spouses without DS. Most couples lived in an environment closely and consistently supported by nearby family and advocates.

### 13.7.3 Parenting

Little information exists on parenting abilities of individuals with DS, possibly because parents with DS are rare. The issue of parenting as a right of mentally disabled persons is a controversial one; many feel that child-rearing is a skill too demanding for those with DS. Some literature on child abuse reflects the complexity, controversial nature, and negative history of the adequacy of parenting by individuals with mental retardation (Tymchuk 1992). Others, like Giovanna Nigro, view such potential parents quite differently:

> I know some mildly retarded couples who are raising happy healthy children. Their children are no worse off than the hundreds of thousands of children born to families of marginal people, not designated retarded, whose limitations are known to us all and who are sometimes classified as 'culturally deprived'. The children of these retarded couples are, in fact, better off by far, for the retarded parents know they have deficiencies and know they must avail themselves of professional advice. (Nigro 1975, p.134.)

While this statement may seem overly sanguine, it reminds us that there are no simple answers for the retarded individual seeking to become a parent.

## 13.8 Contraception

There is diminished use of the healthcare system for gynaecological care and reproductive issues in women with DS (Elkins *et al.* 1987). While it is recommended that all DS females have a baseline gynaecological examination between 17 and 20 years of age (Cohen 1992), this recommendation is followed infrequently by both physicians and parents as well as others caring for individuals with developmental disabilities. The frequency of repeat examinations depends in part on whether the woman is sexually active (Elkins *et al.* 1987; Cohen 1992).

Contraception is a major concern of parents of individuals with DS. How many individuals with DS are sexually active is not known. In the general US population, the mean age for first sexual intercourse is 14.6 years for females and 13.9 years for males (Blum *et al.* 1988).

While some parents are quite verbal about their concerns, thoughts and fears, many are not comfortable mentioning the subject to caregivers. Thus, providers need to initiate structured, supportive and non-judgmental discussions and informative sharing. Professionals should not conclude that silence from parents means that fears and concerns do not exist and that information has been provided and understood.

Over 70% of females with DS ovulate and thus are fertile at some point (Stearns *et al.* 1960; Scola and Pueschel 1992; Tricomi *et al.* 1964). Contraception, therefore, should be a consideration for some adolescent and adult DS females. There are no forms of contraception that are totally contra-indicated in Down's syndrome (Schwab 1992); however, contraceptive choice should be made considering an individual's cognitive and behavioural status.

Contraceptives currently available include male and female condoms, spermicidal foams and gels, and oral contraceptives (OCP) including combined and progesterone 'minipill' forms. Other contraceptive methods are the diaphragm, cervical cap, vaginal sponge, IUD, Norplant, and intramuscular Depo-Provera. In the non-DS population, the most frequently used methods include combination OCPs, the progesterone minipill and IUDs (Laros 1993).

Barrier methods that require application at each coitus may not be practical for individuals with DS who may require supervision in using the devices (Elkins 1990). Some women with DS may be able to comply with a daily OCP regimen; others may need supervision. Of course, non-barrier methods do not promote sexually transmitted disease prevention. Human immunodeficiency virus (HIV) has been reported in the mentally retarded population. Obviously, other sexually transmitted diseases including syphilis, chlamydia, herpes, hepatitis B and gonorrhoea need to be considered in any sexually active individual regardless of disability (Kastner *et al.* 1989).

Contra-indications to oral contraceptive use in DS are the same as those in women without DS and include a history of thromboembolic disease, liver disease, breast cancer and dysfunctional uterine bleeding during pregnancy. Relative contra-indications or concerns are the presence of cardiac abnormalities, the use of anti-convulsant medications, certain antibiotics or griseofulvin, and unstable thyroid function. The most commonly prescribed oral contraceptives in the general female population are *OrthoNovum 135, Ovcon 35, Ortho Novum 777* and *Triphasil. Lo-Ovral* may be considered for females with DS who have oral contraceptive-related amenorrhea (Laros 1993).

Recent FDA approvals of *Medroxyprogesteron (DMPA)* and *Norplant* may be useful to the woman with DS who is unable or unwilling to comply with oral contraceptive treatment. DMPA is an effective contraceptive; after one use, at least 50% of women are amenorrheic (Laros 1993). Intramuscular injections of DMPA are given every three months; its contraceptive effect may be longer (Edgerton 1993). Parents and caretakers report simplified management of menstrual hygiene. An annual series of four quarterly injections costs about $200 per year (Laros 1993).

*Norplant* is a progestin-impregnated plastic implant, inserted subcutaneously into upper arm tissue. It is effective for about five years, but can be removed sooner (Laros 1993). Most common side effects include irregular vaginal bleeding. As with DMPA, there is no sexually transmitted disease prevention. Implant and insertion may cost $300 –$400 (Laros 1993). Some of the initial enthusiasm for *Norplant* has decreased with time. In those individuals with side effects, removal may be more complicated than insertion, resulting in discomfort and added expense.

Surgical sterilization, including laparoscopic tubal ligation as well as total abdominal hysterectomy, is extremely controversial. The procedures have a negative past history and frequently require informed consent, as well as involvement by the patient, if possible, in the decision-making process. The paperwork required before surgery may be long and complex. In most cases, the final decision to proceed may require a Human Subjects Committee review. In 1988, the American College of Obstetrics and Gynecologists Committee on Ethics issued a statement to guide physicians reviewing sterilization issues (American College of Obstetrics and Gynecologists Committee on Ethnics 1988). One must always consider that the young woman with DS may have medical problems which could increase her risk of anaesthetic-related morbidity and mortality (Elkins 1990).

Obtaining surgical sterilization for a daughter with DS may be an expensive, emotionally draining, and frustrating experience for parents. There are numerous parental accounts of obstacles and frustrations encountered while obtaining a surgical sterilization for their mentally disabled daughter. A few parents recount 6–7 years of paperwork and legal procedures, particularly in cases where human rights groups/attorneys have taken on the case as a legal project.

## 13.9 HIV Infection

HIV infection in developmentally disabled individuals was reported by Kastner *et al.* as early as 1989. It is difficult to estimate the HIV positivity rate in mentally disabled people, because the use of mental disability and other disabilities as descriptive variables are not included in HIV reporting statistics. Marchetti *et al.* (1990) surveyed 50 states in an attempt to estimate the extent of HIV infection among developmentally disabled adults. Of the 44 states responding, there were 28 individual and institutional caregivers who identified persons having asymptomatic HIV, two as having AIDS-related complex, and one as having full-blown AIDS. HIV-positive individuals were also identified in community based programmes. In total, 45 individuals in eleven states were identified as having HIV infection (Marchetti *et al.* 1990).

Risk behaviours for HIV transmission appear to be the same as those in the general population, i.e., heterosexual activity, homosexual activity and contaminated blood transfusions. In the general population, the ratio of asymptomatic to symptomatic individuals is about 1:10; in the institutionalized population with developmental disabilities, it is 1:8 (Simonds and

Rogers 1992). Communication and cognitive deficits, as well as this group's increased vulnerability to sexual abuse, may make clinical screening for HIV risk difficult (Schor 1987; Kastner *et al.* 1989). The incidence of sexual abuse in developmentally delayed males is unknown. By some investigations based on physical examination, it may be as high as 37% in females (Elvik *et al.* 1990). In the general population by comparison, 14% of females and 2% of males have been reported sexually abused (Blum *et al.* 1988).

## 13.10 Summary

The development of sexuality and of appropriate sexual behaviour of the individual with DS is not only a developmental process of DS individuals but also of society. People with DS need individualized instruction and support to develop appropriate social and sexual behaviour. If services are not provided, many potential, positive things will not occur. The person with DS who displays inappropriate sexual behaviour may represent his own community's failure to recognize and nurture his sexuality.

Medical knowledge and care of individuals with DS have greatly expanded and improved. The medical care of sexual function should be no exception. Routine medical care including urological and gynaecological care should be available to all individuals with DS. Contraception and methods to prevent sexual abuse should be discussed with the individual and his or her parents.

Sexuality may mean different things to different people with DS, from affectionate touching to marriage and children. Individuals with DS have the right to develop and express their sexuality in an emotionally satisfying and socially appropriate manner. Openness, research, resource identification, education, and individualized services are all needed to provide this opportunity.

## References

American College of Obstetrics and Gynecologists Committee on Ethnics (1988) Committee opinion: Sterilization of women who are mentally handicapped (No.63). Washington DC, USA.

Benda CE (1969) Down Syndrome: Mongolism and its management. New York: Grune and Stratton.

Blum RW, Geer L, Hutton L, McKay C, Resnick MD, Rosenwinkel K, and Song Y (1988) The Minnestoa adolescent health survey. Minnesota Medicine 71: 143–5.

Bovicelli L, Orsini LF, Rizzo N, Montacuti V and Bocchetta M (1982) Reproduction in Down syndrome. Obstetrics and Gynecology 59: 135–75.

Cohen WT (1992) Preventive medicine checklist Ohio/Western Pennsylvania: Down Syndrome Network.

Coleman M (1992) Medical care in Down Syndrome: A preventive medicine approach. New York: Dekker.

Edgerton RB (1993) The Contraception report. Some socio-cultural research considerations. In FF de la Cruz and GD Laveck (Eds.) Human sexuality and the mentally retarded, pp. 240–63 New York: Brunner/Mazel.

Edwards J (1988) Sexuality, marriage, and parenting for persons with Down syndrome. In SM Pueschel, The young person with Down syndrome, pp. 187–204, Baltimore MD: Brookes.

Elkins TE (1990) Gynecologic Care. In SM Pueschel and JK Pueschel (Eds.) Biomedical concerns in persons with Down syndrome, pp. 131–46, Baltimore: Brookes.

Elkins TE, Spinnado J and Muram D (1987) Sexuality and family interaction in Down syndrome: Parental report. Journal of Psychosomatic Obstetrics and Gynecology 6: 81–5.

Elvik SL, Berkowitz CD, Nicholas E, Lipman JL and Inkelis SH (1990) Sexual abuse in the developmentally disabled: Dilemmas of diagnosis. Child Abuse and Neglect 14: 497–502.

Goldstein H (1988) Menarche, menstruation, sexual relations and contraception of adolescent females with Down syndrome. European Journal of Obstetrics and Gynaecologic Reproduction Biology 27: 343–9.

Hsiang YH, Berkovitz GD, Bland GL, Migeon CJ and Warren AC (1987) Gonadal function in patients with Down syndrome. American Journal of Medical Genetics 27: 449–58.

Kastner TA, Nathanson R, Marchetti A and Pincus S (1989) HIV infection and developmental services for adults. Mental Retardation 27: 229–32.

Kingsley J and Levitz M (1994) Count us in. Growing up with Down syndrome, Orlando FL: Harcourt Brace.

Koller H, Richardson SA and Katz M (1988) Marriage in a young adult mentally retarded population. Journal of Mental Deficiency Research 32: 93–102.

Lang DJ, Van Dyke DC, Heide F and Lowe PL (1986) Hypospadias and urethral abnormalities in Down syndrome. Clinical Pediatrics 26: 40–2.

Laros A (1993) Adolescent Gynecology Presentation. Unpublished Manuscript, University of Iowa, Iowa City, USA.

Marchetti A, Nathanson R, Kastner T and Owens R (1990) AIDS and state developmental disabilities agencies: A national survey. American Journal of Public Health 80: 54–6.

McCoy EE (1991) Endocrine function in Down syndrome. In IT Lott and EE McCoy (Eds.) Down Syndrome advances in medical care, pp. 71–82, New York: Wiley-Liss.

Monat-Haller RK (1992) Understanding and expressing sexuality, Baltimore MD: Brookes.

Myers BA and Pueschel SM (1991) Psychiatric disorders in a population with Down syndrome. Journal of Nervous and Mental Disease 179: 609–13.

Nigro G (1975) Sexuality in the handicapped: Some observations on human needs and attitudes. Rehabilitation Literature 36: 202–5.

Pueschel SM and Bier JAB (1992) Endocrinologic aspects. In SM Pueschel and JM Pueschel (Eds.) Biomedical concerns in persons with Down syndrome, pp. 259–72, Baltimore MD: Brookes.

Pueschel SM, Orson JM, Boylan JM and Pezzullo JC (1985) Adolescent development in males with Down syndrome. American Journal of Diseases of Children 139: 236–9.

Rani AS, Jyothi A, Reddy PP and Reddy OS (1990) Reproduction in Down syndrome. International Journal of Gynecology and Obstetrics 31: 81–6.

Schor DP (1987) Sex and sexual abuse in developmentally disabled adolescents. Seminars in Adolescent Medicine 3: 1–7.

Schwab WE (1992) Sexuality and Community Living in Down Syndrome: Advances in Medical Care, New York: Wiley-Liss.

Scola PS and Pueschel SM (1992) Menstrual cycles and basal body temperature curves in women with Down syndrome. Obstetrics and Gynecology 79: 91–4.

Sheridan R, Lierena J, Natkins S and Debenham P (1989) Fertility in a male with trisomy 21. Journal of Medical Genetics 26: 294–8.

Simonds RJ and Rogers MF (1992) Epidemiology of HIV in children and other populations. In AC Crocker, HJ Cohen and TA Kastner (Eds.) HIV infection and developmental disabilities, pp. 5–13, Baltimore MD: Brookes.

Smith GR and Berg JM (1976) Down's Anomaly, New York: Churchill-Livingstone.

Stearns PE, Droulard KE and Sahhar FH (1960) Studies bearing on fertility of male and female mongoloids. American Journal of Mental Deficiency 65: 37–41.

Tricomi V, Valenti C and Hall JE (1964) Ovulatory patterns in Down syndrome. American Journal of Obstetrics and Gynecology 89: 651–6.

Tymchuk AJ (1992) Predicting adequacy of parenting by people with mental retardation. Child Abuse and Neglect 16: 165–78.

Walker-Hirsch L and Champagne MP (1992) Circles III : Safer ways. In AC Crocker HJ Cohen and TA Kastner (Eds.) HIV infection and developmental disabilities, pp. 147–58, Baltimore MD: Brookes.

# Part Six: Integration

# 14 School Integration for Down's Syndrome Children: Policies, Problems and Processes

MICHAEL BEVERIDGE

## 14.1 Down's Syndrome Children in a Changing Context

Down's syndrome children are now being studied to see if their development can be accelerated to such a point that they can lead productive and relatively normal lives. This is a change from earlier views of children with Down's syndrome (DS) as ineducable and unable to acquire life skills. Currently the important questions are a) How we can meet their learning requirements appropriately; b) How research can be of use; and c) How resources and facilities can be provided for their special needs. Furthermore, in the economically developed countries, for example those represented by the OECD, government policies now favour an integrated education system; and the research emphasis has changed from studying whether integration is effective to determining the best ways of achieving it.

Recent OECD reports provide important evidence as to the way different countries are engaging in this process of implementation (OECD 1994a, b). These reports indicate that despite agreements in policy there are considerable differences in practice between countries.

Changes in views of normal education have also influenced attitudes towards integration. The main purpose of education is no longer seen to be the production of elite groups. It is now seen as a preparation for adult life for all pupils, and has broadened from a purely academic perspective to include a wide range of functional skills. Making this connection between the world of work and the school curriculum allows us to take account of special populations and to examine the lifestyles to which they might be appropriately fitted. Consequently the DS population are considered as having those rights of access and opportunity which extend to the population as a whole. All decisions and policy initiatives taken concerning Down's syndrome must now be subject to scrutiny by the same value system as that by which we evaluate educational policy for the normal population.

Down's syndrome children are no longer regarded as non-developing persons who require very limited provision throughout their lives. It is no longer acceptable to allocate these children to a separate life which accepts their entry condition as their final state. We now know that DS children respond to education if learning opportunities are appropriate, and that there are many ways in which they can lead lives which are no different from the non-DS population.

However, for Down's syndrome, as for all of us, 'living normally' requires adjustment by both oneself and society. We now recognize that modern society contains many subcultural groups. Communities are coming to understand that they have inherent diversity, with special groups who require careful understanding. But recognizing that these groups exist is not enough, their needs must also be considered. This shift of emphasis has highlighted the point that schools are now required to show that *they* cannot meet the needs of a DS child where, previously, they stated that the *child* could not adjust to the requirements of the school. Schools have to accommodate to many changes in the school population. Dealing with the special needs of DS children, while raising many important issues of practicality, is consistent with the principle that schools cannot remain static and independent of societal change.

It should also be remembered that DS children are by no means the only ones experiencing difficulties in learning, though they may present the school system with particular problems. Integrating DS children may require examination of the school system as a whole, but they can no longer be excluded merely on grounds of learning difficulty. As we shall see, their needs are probably best met through continuity of special provision which requires collaboration and planning across several parts of the education system. This is exactly the kind of change which is difficult to implement as it requires collaboration between different sectors and institutions, such as primary and secondary schools.

## 14.2 Down's Syndrome Children's Rights and the Law

It is now clear that legislating for integration does not abolish the controversy that surrounds it. For example, while US Public Law 94–142 requires a continuum of alternative educational placements, Biklen (1989) has suggested that this merely leads to children having to meet certain criteria in order to progress to a more 'normal' environment.

To overcome this problem, Sailor (1989) proposed the 'least restrictive environment' principle for selecting pupils' school context. This was defined as 'the environment which provides the least restriction on pupil involvement with others'. But even such a simple guideline has hidden pitfalls.

It has often been assumed that the local comprehensive school would be the obvious choice to satisfy this condition. Some authors, e.g. Lipsky and Gartner (1989) regard this solution as paying too much attention to the physical setting and less to the support services that people require to be integrated into communities. However, if one is legislating for children's rights this is exactly the kind of issue which needs clarification through discussion, consultation and, in some cases, legal action. It is very unlikely that the interpretation of the laws surrounding integration will remain unchanging or unchallenged in the years to come.

Associated with the legal issues are the dilemmas of 'labelling' pupils with special needs. The potential negative effects of labelling have been extensively researched and discussed since the early 1960s (Jenkinson 1993). There is much evidence on the positive effects of positive labels on the self-esteem of children. It is also clear that the opposite can and does occur (Wang and Baker 1986; Chapman 1988). However, educational research requires identification and description of special populations. Some categorization and labelling is necessary to carry out high quality scientific research and to target appropriate intervention strategies.

Not all families and children are willing to accept potential 'stigmatization through labels' so as to benefit from special education provision. Many social and psychological forces work powerfully in the direction of stigmatizing small and unusual groups of people. We need to find ways of both understanding and acting to the benefit of small sections of the population without engaging in a comparison process with ideal types of 'normal' person to which we believe the majority belong. More important perhaps is the possibility that freeing ourselves from prejudice allows a more objective investigation of the educational possibilities for special groups including DS children, without having to engage in too much unpopular affirmative action.

## 14.3 Types of Integration and Ways of Implementing Them

In the UK, the Warnock Committee (DES 1978) distinguished between locational, social and functional integration. The independence of these categories is shown by examples of integration in which children are located in the same school but receive a different curriculum taught by different teachers (Williams 1993). Such children may or may not encounter each other socially and their curricula may be such as to deliver different functional skills.

In the US, locational integration is defined as having 79% of time in an ordinary school. However, it is easy to adopt arbitrary criteria concerning location, but social and functional integration is much more difficult to define. The evaluation of integration programmes is beset by difficulties in defining adequate methods for measuring these two integration types. Many integration programmes aim for social and functional integration but measures of their success have been difficult to identify.

Cutting across these issues is the general pattern of normal education in which homogeneous groupings appear in many schools at all levels of ability. As Booth (1983) points out, the segregation of pupils with severe learning difficulties is no different in principle to the common practice of placing children together according to ability. It is clear, however, that there is a major issue here concerning school organization. Of particular consequence are the resource issues associated with the identification of particular groups and the social identity of the groups themselves. Equally important is the flexibility of the segregation process, i.e., how easy it is for children to move between groups according to performance. This is closely connected to the organization of the school curriculum. In the UK, the new National Curriculum should allow pupils' work to be evaluated on a continuum of difficulty, but it is currently unclear as to how this is working out in practice.

Where integration programmes have been implemented we see, typically, a continuum of provision using some or all of four main components (Jenkinson 1993). These are:

1 Integrated classes in which children with special needs are taught as part of ordinary classes of pupils;
2 Cooperating classes where ordinary and special classes are together part of the time;
3 Classes of children with special needs taught by special teachers in ordinary schools;
4 Support within the normal school from peripatetic teachers with particular skills in teaching special needs children.

These components of integration belong to the school system, but it must be remembered that issues such as special class *v.* regular class may be less crucial for DS children than the development of community based approaches. At the very least, school integration that is not accompanied by attempts to integrate special needs children within their local communities is very likely to fail.

There is little research that has attempted to make comparative evaluation of the four components indicated above. However, a study in Austria is currently attempting such an evaluation (OECD 1994b). It is clear, however, that when countries implement integration programmes they find themselves developing a continuum of provision which leads inevitably to reconsideration of the role of special schools. For example, the above OECD study shows that Canada, Finland, Ireland, Italy, Norway, and Spain are actively considering a change of role of special schools, e.g., in Norway 40 boarding special schools are being emptied and transformed into specialist support centres.

## 14.3 The Process of Integration

The integration process for both special schools and individual children should begin with brief but regular visits. In fact, Jowett (1989) found that 80% of schools for children with Specific Learning Difficulties (SLD) already have links with regular schools. These exchange visits allow identification of the needs of both child and school. They help to ensure that the transition process is smooth and the inevitable fears and anxieties on both sides are reduced. The timescale for integration may need to be long so that all the component parts leading to success can be in place. It must be associated with a firm commitment to integration, with clear decisions and guidelines. A recent study in New Brunswick shows how this planning process influences the success of integration policies (OECD 1994a).

Integration involves not only schools but also policy makers, agencies, local communities, families and students. As such, the considerable planning and preparation should focus on multiple-level system change (Hamre-Nietupski *et al.* 1990). However, within this complex systems approach we should not ignore the role of individual, highly-motivated initiators. People with commitment to integration are essential to the successful monitoring of the change process. All social change is difficult and requires energy and commitment which draws on the vision of individuals.

There are a number of reasons why DS children may require learning experiences which differ from other students.

1 They may engage in slower learning of the same content;
2 They may learn the same content very superficially;
3 They may be selective in what they learn;
4 They may benefit from different ways of accessing learning materials;
5 They may require additional teaching;
6 Alternative content may be required.

One particular issue concerning curriculum planning for DS children is the extent to which the 'developmental curriculum based on normal progression in learning' provides an appropriate model. This can lead DS children to be permanently locked into learning skills which are appropriate only for very young children. This in itself can reinforce stigmatization. The well-documented difficulties experienced by DS children in transferring and generalizing skills suggest that instructions should be directly in areas of immediate value. DS children are also likely to acquire some skills at a slower rate and are much more likely to lose them if they are not practised (see Nadel, Chapter 2). Consequently, the curriculum needs to be broken down into smaller steps and be more carefully sequenced. In addition, teachers need to be able to manage the reinforcing of contingencies as well as carry out the individual task analyses required. There is thus good reason for providing special support to assist teachers in classrooms. All of these issues point to the need for research into how disruptive these changes might be for ordinary classes.

The normal school curriculum encourages increasing specialization of students as they move up through the school system. Hence secondary education poses far greater problems for integration than primary education. Secondary schools tend to be staffed with subject specialists concerned with knowledge rather than overall approaches to learning. Not surprisingly, a growing trend has been noted for students with DS to drift towards special schools when they reach secondary education. Jenkinson (1993) has noted a similar trend in Australia. Clearly the key factors are the age at which students are asked to specialize and the attitudes and skills of subject teachers in secondary schools.

## 14.4 'Whole School' Issues in Integration Programmes

As was indicated earlier, integration will only be successful for substantial numbers of children if a systemic approach is adopted during what may be a lengthy change process. A crucial element is the school as an entity in itself. To ignore the school as a community is very likely to bring about difficulties and contradictions for the pupils with special needs. Despite the teacher-time involved in whole school approaches, the long-term viability of change requires that the school community supports and actively creates an appropriate new culture to accommodate DS children.

This approach will involve the school in examining attitudes and beliefs which concern current students as well as new students with special needs. The school will be required to recognize social and life skills as well as academic achievement, and this must apply to all children if functional integration is to be achieved. The school must examine its standard programmes of education as they affect individual children, perhaps in more detail and with more objectivity than previously. In association with this, the goals of education for all children will probably need to be made more explicit. Identifying alternative and valid school career paths for individuals has long been part of the way special needs children have been taught. The same principle can and should be usefully applied to the student population as a whole. All of these issues carry with them important implications for the staff training and professional development of teachers.

In the UK, the first national in-service training course for teachers within integrational schools run by the Open University had five provisional aims:

1 To update teachers on the new methods of direct teaching of pupils with learning difficulties;
2 Introduction to the process of cooperative teaching through practical and theoretical methods;
3 Methods of supporting children with temporary difficulties;
4 Consultancy work with mainstream colleagues;
5 Organizing and running in-service training for main stream colleagues.

In general, professional development courses leading to integration programmes have been shown to require a comprehensive package including theory, awareness raising material, information and practical techniques. For teachers to benefit from the necessary experiential training process they must have opportunities for practice and feedback and time release for reflection and planning. This work must be supported through integration with other teachers, visits to schools and establishing formal networks to exchange ideas. As indicated earlier, all this must be supported by the head teacher's endorsement and whole-school training and commitment.

## 14.5 Support for Teachers

An important and successful element of many integration programmes concerns additional support for the classroom teacher. However, it is clear that merely adding another adult to a classroom is not in itself likely to be beneficial. Additional specialist support requires careful planning, decision making and record keeping. Support teachers should not just focus on children with special needs, they should be able to take the whole class, giving the class teacher the chance to observe special needs pupils in action. This leads to better planning for the whole class. An important aspect of the planning process must include ensuring that resources and materials are available to teachers and children when needed.

Integration programmes will require the help of external support staff. Psychologists, speech and language pathologists and counsellors have a crucial role in the success of integration programmes. However, these external services must work towards helping teachers to cope themselves and not depend on outside agencies: they have a crucial professional development role. Otherwise, external service staff can find themselves exercising a gate-keeping function and, when teachers are overwhelmed by problems of integration, reasons for excluding special needs children are sought. Such a situation requires careful handling and can place external staff in a difficult position.

The recent OECD reports show how interschool links can be beneficial in establishing school networks to help disseminate good practice through regional meetings of teachers and advice centres; examples of schools supporting each other in this way are found in the Netherlands, Canada and Switzerland. A Belgian study has shown how members of a parents' association formed in the 1970s have linked with the professional staff of a child guidance centre to establish a support service to aid communication between schools. An Australian programme brought teachers together in workshops on 'action research', focusing on children within their classes. There, the teachers plan a programme which is then implemented, evaluated and returned back to the workshop where the process is repeated.

## 14.6 Pupil Ratios

One of the questions raised by parents and schools concerns the number and ratio of special needs children that can be accommodated within a normal school. The number of students with learning difficulties in one school influences how much special service provision can be justified. Thomason and Arkle (1980) and Gartner and Lipsky (1987) suggest that in order to justify adequate support services within a school, the percentage of SLD children can be as high as 25%. However, a notional upper limit must exist otherwise integration would recreate special schools on a larger scale. Empirical evidence on the ratio question is difficult to discover because of the many differing definitions of special needs which exist across different countries. However, a study in the Netherlands (OECD 1994) which examined a child population of 2789 with a pupil–teacher ratio of 21:1, had successfully integrated 260 children with special needs, of whom 88 would otherwise have attended special schools. This study does seem to provide workable guidelines for urbanized populations.

Special schools themselves can have an important role in supporting special needs children in ordinary schools. For example, one UK school ran outreach services to support 189 children in ordinary school in addition to its own 120 children. Some teachers in the ordinary schools were reciprocally attached to the special school (OECD 1994a).

## 14.7 Attitudes to Integration and Social Learning

Research has tended to focus on the social and attitudinal aspects of integration rather than investigating long-term learning outcomes for individual students. This is perhaps not surprising because the DS population has long been subject to prejudicial views concerning their educative potential and general social behaviour, and the change to a policy of integrated education requires such attitudes to be confronted and overcome if the new approaches are to be effective. Research has also investigated self-esteem and changes in self-concept associated with the move to integrated environments (Chapman 1988). Such work has close links with the work on normal children indicating the connection between self-concept and educational achievement.

The move to integrate DS children requires more than just an absence of prejudice. Success requires positive attitudes because the change process itself requires extra effort. DS children require highly motivated teachers to implement integrated educational programmes, especially because most systems of integration make teachers more open to scrutiny, for example, by the presence of teaching assistants in the classroom. The relatively low instance of DS children means that most members of the community are unaware of their difficulties and their educational potential. Integration provides ordinary people with the benefits of learning about DS children, but the existence and effects of initial prejudice cannot be ignored.

Not all parents favour integration. OECD reports from Denmark, Ireland, the Netherlands and Norway refer to some parents preferring segregated settings. They often suspect integration as being an economic measure – not unreasonably, in some cases. Hegarty and Pocklington (1981) show that parents tend to favour segregation if they have not experienced integration. Furthermore, parents of other children in reception classes have views which are not always supportive. They worry about the teacher's attention being drawn towards special needs children. Interestingly, children may well be more favourably disposed to integration than either their parents or teachers, as indicated by an attitude questionnaire in 48 Irish schools. Certainly the parents of DS children in normal schools have reason to be concerned about the expertise available for their children.

Problems of stigmatization of DS children may well arise in the normal school environment. As well as the more overt signs, such as name calling and bullying, stigmatization can occur in subtle ways. Even children who receive additional support in ordinary classrooms can be made to feel inferior. There is a strong tendency for normal children to treat DS children differently, even when prejudice or negative attitudes disappear. For example, their language tends to be modified as if they were talking to younger children. These subtle aspects of the social environment and their effects are not currently well understood.

One important negative feature of segregated schools is the absence of appropriate role models for DS children (Beveridge 1992). Teaching DS children to model their social behaviour on ordinary children has been shown to be effective (Strain and Odom 1988). Given the emphasis in the curriculum for special needs children on social and life skills, this positive effect of integration is perhaps the single most important reason for bringing DS children into the ordinary school. Less often noted, but perhaps equally important, is the way normal children can learn consideration of others by seeing teachers adjust to the special needs of DS children. However, merely placing DS children in normal schools is unlikely on its own to be the most effective procedure. Deliberate strategies need to be used to encourage social integration. These involve the location of special classes, time-tabling, common curricular activities and voluntary peer tutoring. Each of these should be organized to maximize contact between DS and normal children.

Roth and Nardi (1987) have shown that merely having special classes in ordinary schools does not increase social interchange. This problem was recognized early on in the Madison High School Integration Programme (Gruenewald and Schroeder 1981). This programme had a functional emphasis in which integration focused on non-academic and extra-curricular components. Special attention was taken to ensure a sharing of assemblies, cafeteria, passageways, library and other amenities. The SLD students were taught functional living skills with regular and special teachers cooperating in joint programmes.

## 14.8 Economic Issues

In the US in 1985–86 the average cost per child of special education was two to three times that of ordinary education. The range was 1.9–10.6 depending on the disability. In 1989 in the Netherlands, the average cost was approximately four times as high in special education. These general figures do not take account of integration or non-integration. However, they show how, in an integrated environment, resource issues are inevitably going to be prominent. The 1994 OECD study indicated that special school placements cost between two to five times more than in integrated settings. It is perhaps no wonder that many governments regard integration as an appropriate education policy, and similarly parents may be justified in worrying that integration loses resources previously earmarked for their children. Current moves towards educational 'quasi markets', in which funding for schools follows the students, could make DS children attractive resource generators. However, there is little guarantee that once a resource has entered a school budget that it would be spent in the education of the children with whom it is associated (Barrow 1995). Only very clear legislation as to the resource allocation procedures could ensure appropriate use of special needs money.

The way in which resource allocation is organized within the educational system influences the way decisions concerning integration are taken. In England and Italy formal multi-disciplinary assessment of children brings additional resources from both regional and national sources. However, this way of allocating money leaves little guarantee that the appropriate range of in-school services will be available for DS children.

## 14.9 Problems and Conclusions

The recent OECD reports show a number of successful education programmes operating across many different countries. They have also identified a number of common difficulties. There is often resistance by special educators whose career paths have separated them from the normal education system and whose approach to the education process is often very different to the normal class teacher. There is also a tendency for multi-disciplinary services set up to support integration programmes to be concerned with diagnosis and placement rather than giving help with teaching efforts. Even when efforts are made to train school personnel to resolve difficulties referrals to outside agencies continue to be made in 25% of cases (Janney and Meyer 1990).

Lastly, health issues that surround the DS pupils are not usually faced by normal schools (Wolraich 1986). Anxieties about health, concerning responsibility and care, require careful handling within the change process.

Despite these difficulties, a variety of integrated education programmes for DS children is being successfully implemented. However, research into the effects of these programmes on learning outcomes is sparse. In general, the current view is optimistic that integration will enhance the lives of the DS population, but, as this chapter has argued, great care must be taken to improve and maintain the provision which arises through integration policies.

## References

Barrow MJ (1995) The education market. Paper presented at ESRC Seminar on Quasi-Markets. School for Policy Studies, University of Bristol.

Beveridge MC (1992) Social cognition and the Communicative Environment of Mentally Handicapped People. In M Beveridge, G Conti-Ramsden and I Leudar (Eds) Language and communication in mentally handicapped people, pp.143–53. London: Chapman and Hall.

Biklen DP (1989) Redefining schools. In D Biklen, D Ferguson and A Ford (Eds) Schooling and disability. Eighty-eighth yearbook of the National Society for the Study of Education, pp.19–24. Chicago IL: National Society for the Study of Education.

Booth T (1983) Policies towards segregation. British Journal of Special Education 13: 94–5.

Chapman JW (1988) Learning-disabled children's self concepts. Review of Educational Research 58: 347–71.

Department of Education and Science (1978) Special Educational Needs (Warnock Report). London: Her Majesty's Stationery Office (HMSO).

Gartner A and Lipsky DK (1987) Beyond special education: towards a quality system for all students. Harvard Educational Review 57: 367–95.

Gruenewald LJ and Schroeder RJ (1981) Integration of moderately and severely handicapped students in public schools – concepts and processes. In Centre for Educational Research and Innovation, The Education of the Handicapped Adolescent: Integration in the School, pp.65–85. Paris: Organisation for Economic Cooperation and Development.

Hamre-Nietupski S, Nietupski J and Maurer S (1990) A comprehensive state education agency plan to promote the integration of students with moderate/severe handicaps. Journal of the Association for Persons with Severe Handicaps 15: 106–13.

Hegarty S and Pocklington K (1981) Education pupils with special needs in the ordinary school. Windsor UK: National Foundation for Educational Research in England and Wales NFER-Nelson.

Janney RE and Meyer LH (1990) A consultation model to support integrated educational services for students with severe disabilities and challenging behaviour. Journal of the Association for Persons with Severe Handicaps 15: 186–99.

Jenkinson JC (1993) Correlates of sociometric status among TMR children in regular classrooms. American Journal of Mental Deficiency 88: 332–5.

Jowett S (1989) Links between special and ordinary schools – a study of their prevalence and purpose. European Journal of Special Needs Education 5: 23–4.

Lipsky DK and Gartner A (1989) Building the future. In DK Lipsky and A Gartner (Eds) Beyond separate education for all, pp.255–90. Baltimore MD: Brookes.

OECD (1994a) Active life for disabled youth –Integration in the school. Case studies in integration. Good practice across OECD countries in educating children with special needs in ordinary schoools. Distributed 3 March 1994.

OECD (1994b) Active life for disabled youth – Integration in the school. Special education principles, practice and prospects across OECD countries. Distributed 3 March 1994.

Roth MA and Nardi GA (1987) A comparison of program locations and opportunities for public school students with severe handicaps. Education and Training in Mental Retardation 22: 236–43.

Sailor W (1989) The educational, social and vocational integration of students with the most severe disabilities. In DK Lipsky and A Gartner (Eds) Beyond separate education: Quality education for all, pp.53–74. Baltimore MD: Brookes.

Strain PS and Odom SL (1988) Innovations in the education of preschool children with severe handicaps. In R Horner, L Meyer and HD Frederisks (Eds) Education of learners with severe handicaps, pp.61–98. Baltimore MD: Brookes.

Thomason J and Arkle C (1980) Education the severely/profoundly handicapped in the public schools: A side-by-side approach. Exceptional children 47: 114–22.

Wang MC and Baker ET (1985) Mainstreaming programs: design features and effects. Journal of Special Education 19: 503–21.

Williams P (1993) Integration of students with moderate learning difficulties. European Journal of Special Needs Education 8: 303–19.

Wolraich ML (1986) The consequences for health professionals in mainstreaming handicapped children. In CJ Meisel (Ed) Mainstreaming handicapped children: outcomes, controversies and new directions, pp.149–64. Hillsdale NJ: Erlbaum.

# 15
# Social and Labour Integration of People with Down's Syndrome

JUAN PERERA

## 15.1 Introduction

I end this book with a chapter on the integration of people with Down's syndrome (DS) in society and in work. This is because the incorporation into work of people with DS constitutes the final step towards full participation in the life of their community (Kiernan *et al.* 1989).

Before beginning, it is important to specify a few points. Firstly, assuming a normal distribution of intellectual abilities in Down's syndrome (all subetiologies confounded) with a mean IQ of 47–50 and a standard deviation (SD) of around 8, approximately 68% of DS individuals will fall within the range defined by the IQ ±1 SD, i.e.,50 ±8. Approximately 16% of DS individuals will fall outside this range on either side of the distribution.

Secondly, exceptional cases are frequently presented, in books and articles, but primarily at congresses and in the news media, of individuals who are not typical of Down's syndrome – people who are exceptionally gifted and have had special training facilities not available to everyone. In fact, presenting 'typical cases' is more positive because it serves as an incentive to parents and professionals and because it helps to break down negative attitudes and facilitates the social integration of people with DS.

Thirdly, when we discuss work prospects for people with DS we are talking about competitive work in a market economy. It is obvious, however, that it is very difficult for people with significant mental retardation to be employed in competitive jobs if the economy is not expanding and there is a high rate of unemployment in the 'world of work' (Stark and Goldsbury 1988).

## 15.2 What Sort of People are the DS Individuals Whom We Want to Incorporate in Work or Who are Already Working?

I want to refer to the pattern of normality in Down's syndrome and analyse, firstly, what people with DS are like. This is done in the full knowledge that all generalisations are incorrect, and that special emphasis has been put on the negative aspects in order to try to compensate for them.

### 15.2.1 The cognitive aspects

On scanning through the psychological literature relative to Down's syndrome in the last decade (Berry *et al.* 1984; Carr 1985; Buckley and Sacks 1987; Cicchetti and Beeghly 1990; Cunningham 1995), I have singled out, among other significant elements that affect the cognitive processes of people with DS, the following areas of difficulty:

1 Mental deficiency (average MA is 8–10 years) (Wishart 1992; K. Wisniewski, Chapter 1).
2 Problems in visual and auditory perception (Pueschel 1988).
3 Alterations in the perception of time and space (Cicchetti and Ganiban 1990).
4 Difficulties in short- and long-term memory (see Nadel, Chapter 2).
5 Deficiencies in systems of attention and alertness (see Nadel, Chapter 2).
6 Deficiencies in the mechanisms of information input, processing and integration (Flórez 1995).
7 Failure in the consolidation of acquired knowledge (Hodapp and Mueller 1990).
8 Poor response to stimuli (Perera 1987).
9 Difficulty in the processes of logic, abstraction, deduction and generalization (Hodapp and Mueller 1990).
10 Language and communication problems (Perera and Rondal 1995).

### 15.2.2 Personality and behaviour

Psychologists are often reluctant to describe the personalities of people with DS. Whereas investigations in the medical and genetic fields abound and are highly specialized, in the field of personality there are relatively few published works (but see Caltagirone *et al.* 1990; Pueschel *et al.* 1991; Wootton 1991; Schapiro *et al.* 1992; Cuskelly and Gunn 1993; Seltzer *et al.* 1993).

With regard to employment, the following common denominators

Table 15.1 Tasks to be done – Example: In a greenhouse

1. *To multiply plants*
1.1 Prepare soil
1.2 Sow manually
1.3 Take cuttings and sow them
1.4 Sow mechanically

2 *To Cultivate the Soil*
2.1 Dig soil
2.2 Stake
2.3 Fertilize
2.4 Tend a plant
2.5 Transplant
2.6 Water
2.7 Weed

3 *To protect the plants*
3.1 Clean a plant
3.2 Detect a disease
3.3 Apply a treatment
3.4 Control a treatment

4. *To control a greenhouse*
4.1 Regulate the light
4.2 Regulate the temperature
4.3 Regulate the humidity
4.4 Regulate watering

5 *To maintain a greenhouse*
5.1 Maintain the structure
5.2 Maintain control systems
5.3 Maintain equipment and tools

6 *To prepare for marketing*
6.1 Follow a marketing programme
6.2 Prepare an order
6.3 Prepare and pack the plants

can be found on evaluating the personality and behaviour of a person with DS.

1 Diminished capacity to respond to what is new (fewer interactions with the environment);
2 Diminished capacity to analyse and interpret external events;
3 Lack of responsibility in continuing the effort; diffuse behaviour; increasing resistance to effort;
4 Tendency to depend on older adults and reduced personal autonomy;

Table 15.2 Work Methods and Times for each Task
Example: Place a Seed in a Container

*Sequential operations*

| | *Left hand* | *Right hand* | *Time* |
|---|---|---|---|
| 1. | Place the container in work position | Place the container in work position | 5" |
| 2. | Fill the container with soil | Fill the container with soil | 10" |
| 3. | Hold the container | Take the planting tool | 3" |
| 4. | Hold the container | Make the hole | 3" |
| 5. | Hold the container | Take the seed | 5" |
| 6. | Hold the container | Sow the seed | 5" |
| 7. | Hold the container | Cover the seed with soil | 5" |
| 8. | Place the container on transport trolley | Place the container on transport trolley | 5" |
| | | Total Time | 36" |

Start a new sequence of operations

36" × Container
In 1 hour = 129 Containers
In 1 day = 1032 Containers

Table 15.3 Practical and Theoretical Knowledge Required for each Task
Example: To Sow Manually

**1.2.1** *To Prepare the Bed for Sowing*
- The sieve
- Know how to sieve
- Know how to spread the soil in the container
- Know how to level out
- Know how to estimate humidity
- Know how to humidify

**1.2.2** *To Sow the Seed*
- Know the seeds (characteristics, forms, colours, etc.)
- Know the different forms of manual planting: seed by seed, sprinkling...
- Know how to handle the planting tool

**1.2.1** *To Cover the Seed*
- Know how to distinguish: top/bottom
- Have an idea of depth
- Assimilate the importance of correct depth
- Know the germination conditions

**1.2.4** *To Store the Prepared Containers*
- Know how to stack
- Know how to move containers
- Place them in the proper place

**1.2.5** *To Monitor the Evolution of a Seedbed*
- Know the germination conditions
- Know times of germination
- Know anomalies

5 Lower consciousness of their own limitations (e.g., people with DS often fail to anticipate danger);
6 Low expectancy of success;
7 Lack of initiative;
8 Lack of motivation.

The negative characteristics listed here, that hinder the integration of people with DS into the labour market (Floyd 1995), reveal that both the European Union's policy on employment for the disabled and the organizations representing people with a disabilities, are not meeting the needs of people with DS regarding their incorporation into the 'world of work'.

## 15.3 Training: How Should People with Down's Syndrome be Prepared for Work?

Assuming that people with DS have a minimum, basic and obligatory school training, usually acquired in a special or integrated school, we are faced with an adult subject whose real level of knowledge, acquisitions and abilities are at the level of about the 2nd or 3rd grade in basic education (in the Spanish educational system), but who, in practice, has an average MA of 8–10 years and is ahead or behind in certain areas. This is the base line from which we have to start training people with DS for work and requires 'knowledge of each subject's singularity and diversity' (Perera 1995).

It is obvious that this level of knowledge and ability limits a young person with DS to work that only involves the *execution of simple tasks* which do not require complex intellectual operations or complicated manual dexterity (Perera 1987).

Reports published on people with DS who have been incorporated in work mostly refer to auxiliary jobs in sales, stores, cooking, gardening, hotels, services, assembling, maintenance, packing... always under a certain level of supervision or support (Chigier 1990). This indicates that it is neither practical nor profitable to try to give a young person with DS theoretical professional training for an occupation. It is much more positive to orient training towards specific tasks that offer a real possibility of work.

What sort of training should they be given? Based on my experience, I recommend the following systematic approach. First, identify the job and analyse what is involved; then evaluate the subject's aptitudes and limitations and design an individualized training programme before letting them start the work. The greater the subject's limitations, the more detailed the job analysis and the training programme will have to be.

### 15.3.1 Identification of the job

In order to prepare young people with DS for work, it is fundamental that one first identifies what jobs a community has to offer this type of person: only then should a training programme for these jobs be organized – not the other way round. 'Identify the job' involves negotiating with the firm or with the employers' association and arriving at an agreement which, within a specified period of time, will make it possible for a serious and stable labour relationship to be initiated. There have been too many cases of schemes starting up and then foundering, resulting in frustration and disappointment for all concerned.

### 15.3.2 Job analysis

Each of the tasks to be done needs to be described, grouped and put into sequence. (See Table 15.1 for an example showing the tasks to be done in the cultivation of plants in a greenhouse.) The methods and times to perform each task must be studied in order to economise on effort, to prevent wasted time and to make the work more comfortable and profitable (see Table 15.2). Finally, the minimal knowledge required to execute each task has to be defined (see Table 15.3).

### 15.3.3 Evaluation of each subject's aptitude, limitations and needs

Apart from the job, it is necessary to study the aptitudes, limitations and needs of the individual subject who is going to fill the job. Tests, questionnaires, evaluation scales, social reports, etc. will provide a sound evaluation of the subject's abilities. There are studies (Smith *et al.* 1989) that meticulously analyse these needs. It may be useful to refer to the concept of 'adaptive abilities' (Anastasi 1986), that can be extended to various domains or areas (see Meyers *et al.* 1979; Kamphaus 1987; McGrew and Bruininks 1989; Widaman *et al.* 1991; Widaman *et al.* 1993) and constitute the appropriate basis for this evaluation.

### 15.3.4 Designing an individualized programme

In comparing the demands of the tasks to be done with the subject's abilities and limitations, an individualized training programme can be defined in which objectives, contents, strategies and activities are specified with the aim of preparing and qualifying the subject for work.

### 15.3.5 Opportunity to work

In my experience, the key to success has been giving an individual with DS the opportunity to work in a job for which he or she has been prepared and trained. When given this opportunity, people with DS are capable of gradually adapting themselves better to the work and, what is more interesting, they also become increasingly capable of performing more complex tasks.

## 15.4 Work Alternatives

To give a young person with DS a genuine 'opportunity to work' means offering him or her choices most suited to their capacity, and previous training. What are the main work alternatives?

### 15.4.1 Occupational Centres and protected workshops

Young people with DS who have *severe* physical or mental disabilities usually attend this type of centre. There they are given the opportunity to improve their school abilities and to learn some occupational skills. Preparing people with DS for employment is *not* the main objective of these centres as it is assumed that they do not have the capacity to carry out real jobs – so they are not 'work' centres in the real sense of the word. They are not usually profitable or competitive, nor are they run with entrepreneurial criteria. But these centres fulfil a necessary and important social function. Persons who are occupied there – that is why they are called Occupational Centres – can be there for life. Parents and professionals take on great responsibility if they decide to limit a person with DS to a centre of this type, without giving that person the opportunity to demonstrate his or her capacities and without supplying him or her any other options for work.

### 15.4.2 Special Employment Centres

In Spain, Special Employment Centres constitute the principal labour alternative for people with different types of disabilities and are a real and interesting alternative for people with DS. The centres are run as businesses that compete with entrepreneurial criteria and with all the obligations and rights of firms in the market, but with a section of the permanent workforce made up of people with some kind of disability.

Whether this alternative is more or less normalizing or integrating depends on the number of non-disabled workers, the job being done, the employment services, personal support, and management criteria.

All over the world, people with DS are working, with remarkable satisfaction, in Special Employment Centres or similar centres with corresponding legislation, dedicated to greenhouse cultivation, maintenance of green zones, computers, printing, restoration work etc. It should be mentioned that the failures occurring in such centres are not due to the disabled workers, in our case people with DS, but usually to the lack of a good entrepreneurial structure, proper financing, competitive technology, quality end-products and good management with strictly entrepreneurial criteria.

### 15.4.3 Employment with support

Undoubtedly, Wehman *et al.* (1987) defined one of the most interesting alternatives as: 'A competitive job in integrated environments for those individuals who traditionally have not had this opportunity, using suitably trained employment instructors and promoting systematic training, work development and monitoring services, among others' (p. 180).

In the world of the disabled, the concept of support to increase independence, productivity and integration in the community has experienced renewed interest in recent years (O'Reilly 1988; Schalock and Genung 1993; Schalock 1994a). The support components that appear in current models, are:

- support resources (individual, other people, technological means and services);
- support functions (including teaching, protection, economic planning, behavioural support, help in the home, access and utilisation of the community, and medical attention);
- intensity of the supports supplied (intermittent, limited, extensive, generalized); and
- results of the supports (Schalock 1994b).

The disabled person, i.e., the young person with DS, must be in a full time competitive job or be working no less than twenty hours per week part time. His or her salary must be at least equal to the minimum interprofessional wage, and their post must be fully integrated.

There are different models of 'employment with support' (Verdugo and Jenaro 1993). Among others, I stress the following models:

1 *Competitive employment with support* – Some authors (Powell *et al.* 1990) call it 'individual work'. It involves helping to locate a suitable job, training the disabled candidate in an intensive way, and maintaining continuous support services. A qualified professional establishes a close relationship with the disabled candidate and trains him or her in the actual place of work.

   The disabled person works from the first day and receives wages from the firm. Evaluations of the subject's performance are made daily or weekly. Once the subject has learnt the task properly, the professional gradually reduces the support time. In many cases, colleagues at work or heads of department take over these functions, giving their support to the worker in various situations.

2 *Mobile work groups* – This option has existed for many years. The mobile work groups, also called 'work force teams', comprise from four to six individuals with severe disabilities from a Rehabilitation Centre or an Occupational Centre who do jobs in community outdoor areas (maintenance of public installations, gardening, cleaning trains, etc.). The workers are paid according to their productivity by the organization representing them, which is usually a non-profit making organization. A supervisor accompanies the group all the time and is responsible for the training of the team members. The supervisor is in charge of all facets of the operation, from formalization of insurance and contracts, to training, supervision and maintaining achievements (Bellamy *et al.* 1987). This alternative is of particular interest in small communities and rural areas.
3 *The enclaves* – These are small groups of 6–8 disabled workers who are employed and supervised in businesses and industries by non-disabled workers. A professional carries out continuous supervision in the work-place. The disabled workers can be hired directly by the firm or belong to a non-profit making organization which is responsible for making the arrangements. The enclave members work next to workers without any disability although, in some circumstances, they are grouped in order to facilitate training and assessment. Unlike the above model, where the workers may be working in different places each day or even in different places on the same day, the enclave workers usually work in the same place for a long period of time. Furthermore, with this alternative the workers may receive their wage through the hiring firm. In this model the support is more systematic, continuous, intensive and reliable. Integration is achieved by facilitating interactions with the rest of the employees at rest times, before, and after work, and by means of interactions generated around work (Verdugo and Jenaro 1993).
4 *Small businesses* – Small businesses are usually concerned with activities in commerce, services, manufacturing, production, or assembling of component parts. The two main characteristics of this alternative are, firstly, their small size (maximum 6–8 persons with disability), with an equal number of persons without disability; and secondly, the homogeneity of the work, i.e., all the employees are involved in the same enterprise or task.

   The small firm operates in the same way as any other business, generating employment and paying the employees. It is located in the community which offers possibilities for integration. It is also a particularly interesting alternative for persons demonstrating unsuitable social behaviours, difficulties in verbal communication, etc. (Bellamy *et al.* 1979).

These examples of 'employment alternatives' reveal one thing: no one single method, alternative, or model is ideal. Each individual with

DS (who has unique personal, intellectual characteristics, and concrete aptitudes, limitations and needs) should be placed in the work alternative that will be best suited to his or her apptitudes and needs. And while the ultimate goal is full integration in ordinary work, several steps may be required to reach it. 'Work with support' may encounter many difficulties such as : How is continuous support provided, what happens when it is reduced and who pays for the high cost that this system entails (Parent *et al.* 1991)?

## 15.5 What does 'Work' Mean for People with Down's Syndrome?

Work is a characteristic of adult life for all people, with or without a disability. The type of employment, the wage received, and the opportunities given directly affect the way we perceive ourselves and the way society values us, as well as the degree of freedom we have at the social and economic level (Wehman *et al.* 1987).

Most people aspire to a socially recognized job and a wage that makes it possible to live in comfort (Brolin 1985). Starting from this idea, we can understand the situation of disabled person who is in an Assistance Centre or Occupational Centre, surrounded only by other disabled persons, and without the possibility of doing any paid work. To give this person a job opportunity means not only that he or she will receive a wage, but will also receive recognition of his or her social value within the family and acceptance within the community. Another major benefit is the opportunity to make friends and establish affective links with people who are not disabled (Verdugo and Jenaro 1993).

The wage is an important determinant of the quality of life, both at the emotional and material level. Generally, the better paid a person, the greater the freedom to become established independently in society (Brolin 1985).

'People are what they do' (Montobbio 1992). That is why work gives the individual with DS the capacity to take decisions, transforms him or her into an active person, dignifies his or her economic situation, allows him or her to obtain what he or she wants, and gives him or her security and responsibility (González Yagüe 1990).

Any disabled person whose residual capacity is capable of being converted into useful value must automatically be considered as a 'labour being'. The extraordinary social value of this possibility means that the person with mental retardation (including the person with DS) can be equal to the non-disabled in any job where it is possible for technology to compensate for human limitations (Casas and Miró 1983).

Society's lack of belief in the capacity of disabled people to do a profitable job is the main obstacle to their lack of socio-labour integration

(Núñez 1983). Labour integration is the key to social integration (Kiernan *et al.* 1989).

In a recent study conducted in the Balearic Islands (Asociación Síndrome de Down de Baleares, ASNIMO-SEMPRE VERDE) 16 people with DS were monitored longitudinally during four years in the horticultural sector (greenhouse cultivation). Monthly family and personal records were kept, by the professionals responsible, to evaluate their progress at work as well as their achievements in the field of economic, social and personal autonomy. A brief account of the results follows, in which there was a marked increase (more than 10% in all cases) on the following variables:

A *Variables of a personal type*

1. Self-esteem and self-confidence
2. Feelings of usefulness
3. Definition of own personality traits
4. Personal autonomy
5. Capacity for adapting to what is new
6. Development of abilities
7. Consciousness of the need to make an effort
8. Feeling that the effort is translated into new abilities and results
9. Consciousness of own limitations

B *Variables of a social type*

1. Experience of integration
2. Learning to coexist, share and relate
3. Learning to compete
4. Social status (participation in community life)
5. Security for the future (pension/retirement)
6. Better knowledge of the value of money
7. Increase in level of aspiration

C *Economic variables*

1. Cease to be passive subjects (a burden for society)
2. Become productive subjects

## 15.6 Conclusions

I reach the following conclusions:

1 For adults with Down's syndrome, *it is never too late to learn*, despite the fact that are adults, have not been to school and may present significant impairment.

2 *Non-intervention means augmented retardation.* Put another way, the intervention must be constant, systematic, suitable, and based on personal and effective motivation.
3 *People with DS of any age and condition can work*
- if we study their limitations and their specific capacities and abilities
- if we prepare them properly
- if we adapt the jobs to their specific abilities
- if we give them the opportunity to work on tasks suited to their capacities
- if we give them the necessary support.

4 *Incorporation into work settings can transform the lives of people with DS and integrates them socially.* It turns them into useful members of society. They become more autonomous knowing that their wage is the result of their effort. They share their joys and troubles with their colleagues at work. They improve their quality of life.
5 *They cease to be a burden for society and become productive subjects.* Economically, it is to the advantage of societies to invest in training and job creation for the disabled, among whom are people with DS.
6 *The disabled people have an assured future.* Life expectancy for people with DS has increased considerably (see Rondal, Chapter 7). The parents of some of these young adults will have died already and their brothers or sisters cannot, or do not want to, take care of them. The DS person who is working has more stability and is more likely to become self sufficient, and to be living in an independent way or in small supervised homes, without being a burden on society.

Lastly, it is useful to remember that the brain is not a fixed structure, but is eminently plastic and malleable. It is the base and foundation of behaviour, but behaviour in turn shapes the functioning of the brain (Flórez 1995). For that reason environment and intervention have a decisive influence on the psychological development of the individual, hence Montobbio's statement 'people are what they do' (Montobbio 1992). That is why labour integration leads to better personal maturity and to fuller social integration.

## References

Anastasi A (1986) Intelligence as a quality of behavior. In RJ Sternberg and DK Detterman (Eds) What is intelligence? Contemporary viewpoints on its nature and definition, pp.19–22. Norwood NJ: Ablex.

Bellamy GT, Horner RH and Inman D (1979) Vocational habilitation of severely handicapped adults: a direct service technology. Baltimore MD: University Press.

Bellamy GT, Rhodes L, Mank D and Albin J (1987) Supported employment. A community implementation guide. Baltimore MD: Brookes.

Berry P, Groeneweg G, Gibson D and Brown RI (1984) Mental development in adults with Down syndrome. American Journal of Mental Deficiency 89: 252–6.

Brolin DE (1985) Career education material for exceptional individuals. Career Development for Exceptional Individuals 8: 62–4.

Buckley S and Sacks B (1987) The adolescent with Down's syndrome: Life for teenager and for the family. Portsmouth UK: Portsmouth Down's Syndrome Trust.

Caltagirone C, Nocenti U and Vicari S (1990) Cognitive functions in adult Down's syndrome. International Journal of Neuroscience 54: 221–30.

Carr J (1995) The development of intelligence. In D Lane and B Stratford (Eds) Current approaches to Down's syndrome, pp.167–86. London: Cassell.

Casas J and Miró D (1983) Centros de Empleo Especial. In Plan nacional de empleo, pp.143–67. Madrid: Real Patronato de Prevención y Atención a Personas con Minusvalía.

Chigier E (Ed) (1990) Looking up at Down syndrome.London: Freund.

Cicchetti D and Beeghly M (Eds) (1990) Children with Down Syndrome: a developmental perspective. New York: Cambridge University Press.

Cicchetti D and Ganiban J (1990) The organization and coherence of developmental processes in infants and children with Down syndrome. In R Hodapp, J Burack and E Zigler. Issues in the developmental approach to mental retardation, pp.169–212. New York: Cambridge University Press.

Cunningham CC (1995) Desarrollo psicológico en los niños con síndrome de Down. In J Perera (Ed) Síndrome de Down. Aspectos específicos, p.121-51. Barcelona: Masson.

Cuskelly M and Gunn P (1993) Maternal reports of behavior of siblings of children with Down syndrome. American Journal of Mental Retardation 97: 521–9

Flórez J (1995) Patología cerebral en el síndrome de Down: apredizaje y conducta. In J Perera (Ed) Síndrome de Down. Aspectos específicos, pp. 27–52. Barcelona: Masson.

Floyd L (1995) Disability. Management at work. Siglo Cero 26: 15–20.

González Yagüe A (1990) Propuesta de trabajo sobre Centros Ocupacionales. Comunicación a las I Jornadas sobre Deficiencia y sociedad. Integración laboral del deficiente. Unpublished manuscript: University of Madrid.

Hodapp RM and Mueller E (1990) Applying the developmental perspective to individuals with Down syndrome. In D Cicchetti and M Beeghly (Eds) Children with Down syndrome: A developmental perspective, pp.1–28. New York: Cambridge University Press.

Kamphaus RW (1987) Conceptual and Psychometric issues in the assessment of adaptive behavior. Journal of Special Education 21: 27–35.

Kiernan WE, Schalock RL and Knutson K (1989) Economic and demographic trends influencing employment opportunities for adults with disabilities. In WE Kiernan and RL Schalock (Eds) Economic, industry and disability: A look ahead, pp. 3–16. Baltimore MD: Brookes.

McGrew K and Bruininks R (1989) The factor structure of adaptive behavior. School Psychology Review 18: 64–81.

Meyers C, Nihira K and Zetlin A (1979) The measurement of adaptive behavior. In NR Ellis (Ed) Handbook of mental deficiency: Psychological theory and research, pp.431–81. Hillsdale NJ: Erlbaum.

Montobbio E (1992) La integración social de las personas con discapacidad intelectual: intrumentos, métodos y profesionales. In Síndrome de Down: Para llegar a ser una persona autónoma, pp.415–22. Barcelona: Fundación Catalana para el Síndrome de Down

Nadel L (1996) Consecuencias de las anormalidades cerebrales en el aprendizaje y memoria de las personas con síndrome de Down. In JA Rondal, J Perera and L Nadel (Eds) Down's Syndrome: Psychological, psychobiological and socio-educational perspectives. London: Whurr.

Núñez García-Sarco A (1983) Elaboración. In Plan nacional de empleo,pp.15–50. Madrid: Real Patronato de Prevención y Atención a Personas con Minusvalía.

O'Reilly P (1988) Methodological issues in social support and social network research. Social Science Medicine 26: 863–73.

Parent W, Kregel J, Wehman P and Metzler H (1991) Measuring the social integration of supported employment workers. Vocational Rehabilitation 1: 35–49.

Perera J (1987) Síndrome de Down. Program de acción educativa. Madrid: CEPE.

Perera J (Div) (1995) Síndrome de Down. Aspectos específios. Barcelona: Massan.

Perera J and Rondal JA (1995) Cómo hacer hablar al niño con síndrome de Down y mejorar su lenguaje. Una aproximación psicolingüística. Madrid: CEPE.

Powell TH, Pancsofar EL, Steere DE, Butterworth J, Itzkowitz JS and Rainforth B (1990) Supported employment. Providing integrated employment opportunities for persons with disabilities. New York: Longman.

Pueschel S (1988) Visual and auditory processing in children with Down syndrome. In L Nadel (Ed) The psychobiology of Down syndrome, pp.199–216. Cambridge MA: MIT Press.

Pueschel S, Bernier JC and Pezzullo JC (1991) Behavioural observations in children with Down's syndrome. Journal of Mental Deficiency Research 35: 502–11.

Schalock RL (1994a) Implicaciónes para una investigación de definición, clasificación y sistemas de apoyos de la AAMR de 1992. Siglo Cero 26: 5–13.

Schalock RL (1994b) The assessment of natural supports in community rehabilitation services. In OC Karan and S Greenspan (Eds) Rehabilitation services in the community pp.132–47. New York: Andover Medical Publications.

Schalock RL and Genung LT (1993) Placement from a community-based mental retardation program: a 15-year follow-up. Mental Retardation 98: 400–7.

Schapiro M, Haxby JV and Grady CL (1992) Nature of mental retardation and dementia in Down syndrome: study with PET, CT and neuropsychology. Neurobiology of Aging 13: 723–34.

Seltzer M, Krauss M and Tsunematsu N (1993) Adults with Down syndrome and their aging mothers: Diagnostic group differences. American Journal on Mental Retardation 97: 496–508.

Smith B, Povall M and Floyd M (1989) Managing disability at work. London: City University Resource Centre.

Stark J and Goldsbury T (1988) Analysis of labor and economics: needs for the next decade. Mental Retardation 26: 363–8.

Verdugo MA and Jenaro C (1993) El empleo con apoyo. Una nueva posibilidad laboral para personas con discapacidad. Siglo Cero 24: 5–12.

Wehman P, Moon S, Everson J, Wood W and Barcus J (1987) Transition from school to work. New challenges for youth with severe disabilities. Baltimore MD: Brookes.

Widaman KF, Borthwick-Duffy SA and Little TD (1991) The structure and development of adaptive behavior. In NW Bray (Ed) International Review of Research in Mental Retardation., 17: 1–54. New York: Academic Press.

Widaman KF, Stacy AW and Borthwick-Duffy SA (1993) Construct validity of dimensions of adaptive behavior: a multi-trait–multi-method evaluation. American Journal of Mental Retardation 98: 219–34.

Wisniewski K (1995) Consecuencias de las anormalidades genéticas en la estructura y función del ceretro en las personas con síndrome de Down. In JA Rondal, J Perera and L Nadel (Eds) Down's syndrome: Psychological, psychobiological and socio-educational perspectives. London: Whurr.

Wishart J (1992) El desarrollo de las dificultades de apredizaje en los niños pequeños con síndrome de Down. Para llegar a ser una persona autónoma. Barcelona: Fundación Catalana Síndrome de Down.

Wootton AJ (1991) Offer sequences between parents and young children with Down's syndrome. Journal of Mental Deficiency Research 34: 324–38.

# Concluding Comments

As a way of concluding this long journey into the diversity and complexity of Down's syndrome, we thought that it would be appropriate and of value to reproduce the set of general statements regarding present and future states of research, education and social policy in regard to Down's syndrome, on which the scientific participants in the Palma Symposium agreed.

1. There is a specificity in Down's syndrome deriving from the presence of an extra chromosome 21 (or an essential part of it) which causes significant alterations to the structure and function of the brain and nervous system, and in the learning and behaviour of persons with Down's syndrome.
2. Individual variability is large in Down's syndrome. Consequently, there is a need to approach rehabilitation in a personal and individualized way.
3. As there is no genetic or pharmacological therapy available at present to cure Down's syndrome, rehabilitating efforts must concentrate on educational programmes and favour suitable interactions with the environment.
4. What is known about the specificity of Down's syndrome must be translated into practical facts, therapeutic methods, and concrete measures of intervention aimed at improving the integration of Down's syndrome persons in school, social and professional life.
5. Advances have been observed in the quality of life of persons with Down's syndrome, resulting in:
   - longer life expectancy
   - improved state of health
   - improved intellectual abilities
   - greater skill in carrying out meaningful tasks
   - greater degree of personal autonomy and independence
   - improved integration in school, at work and in society
   - improved understanding on the part of society of the affective and sexual rights of persons with Down's syndrome

6. Recent findings concerning the susceptibility of Down's syndrome persons to develop Alzheimer's disease, confirm the need to design psycho-educational programmes ensuring the stimulation of mental and physical functions, as efficient means of preventing or delaying the appearance of this type of illness and limiting its pathological effects.

*Prof M Beveridge (UK); Prof S Buckley (UK); Prof IG Candel (Spain); Prof M Guralnick (USA); Prof R Hodapp (USA); Prof L Nadel (USA); Prof J Perera (Spain); Prof SM Pueschel (USA); Prof R Remington (U.K.); Prof JA Rondal (Belgium); Prof M Sustrova (Slovakia); Prof D Van Dyke (USA); Prof JG Wishart (UK); Prof H Wisniewski (USA); Prof K Wisniewski (USA).*

Palma de Mallorca, Balearic Islands, February 26th, 1995.

# Name index

# Subject index